TREATMENT OF BRACHIAL PLEXUS INJURIES

Edited by **Vicente Vanaclocha**
and **Nieves Sáiz-Sapena**

Treatment of Brachial Plexus Injuries

http://dx.doi.org/10.5772/intechopen.71238
Edited by Vicente Vanaclocha and Nieves Sáiz-Sapena

Contributors

Claudia Vargas, Fernanda Torres, Bia Ramalho Dos Santos Lima, Cristiane Patroclo, Lidiane Souza, Fernanda Guimarães, José Vicente Martins, Maria Luíza Rangel, Dhiren Ganjwala, Maulin Shah, Jörg Bahm, Bernd Sellhaus, Wissam Elkazzi, Tobias Esser, Frederic Schuind, Chiazor Onyia, Ashok Pillai, Ravi Sankaran, Vicente Vanaclocha, Nieves Sáiz-Sapena

First published in London, United Kingdom, 2019 by IntechOpen
IntechOpen is the global imprint of INTECHOPEN LIMITED, registered in England and Wales, registration number: 11086078, The Shard, 25th floor, 32 London Bridge Street
London, SE19SG – United Kingdom
Printed in Croatia

British Library Cataloguing-in-Publication Data
A catalogue record for this book is available from the British Library

Additional hard and PDF copies can be obtained from orders@intechopen.com

Treatment of Brachial Plexus Injuries, Edited by Vicente Vanaclocha and Nieves Sáiz-Sapena
p. cm.
Print ISBN 978-1-83880-403-9
Online ISBN 978-1-83880-404-6
eBook (PDF) ISBN 978-1-83881-138-9

For EU product safety concerns:
IN TECH d.o.o., Prolaz Marije Krucifikse Kozulić 3, 51000 Rijeka, Croatia,
info@intechopen.com or visit our website at intechopen.com.

Meet the editors

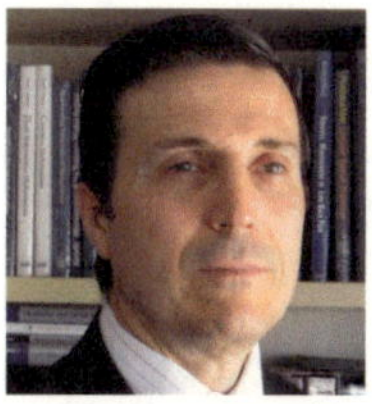

Dr. Vicente Vanaclocha got his medical degree from the University in Valencia and did his training as neurosurgeon in the Hospital affiliated to it. Just from the beginning of his professional career he put a great effort in continuous training. Proof of it is his 15 long term stays in renamed hospital from all over the world and his 182 courses attended. He is always eager to learn and devoted to teach. He has published 75 articles in peer reviewed journals with close to 3000 citations. He has also been involved in humanitarian work in Syria and Egypt. He is a devoted husband and father of three lovely daughters.

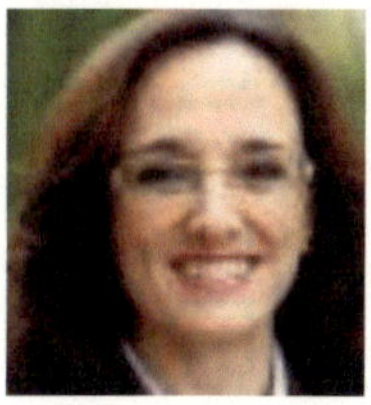

Nieves Saiz-Sapena is Doctor of Medicine from the University of Valencia. She has over 25-year experience in anesthetic management of chronic pain, neuro-oncology, peripheral nerve surgery, and bariatric surgery. She is specialist in Anesthesiology and stay at the Groote Schuur Hospital in Cape Town (South Africa). She was Associate Professor at the University of Navarra, Head of Department of Anesthesiology Hospital San Jaime (Torrevieja, Alicante), Associate Professor Universidad Católica San Vicente Martir, Valencia. Currently she serves as as an editorial board member in several journals.

Contents

Preface

The human shoulder requires a wide range of motion to allow a great variety of movements, among them, throwing objects. This capability is precisely what afforded our ancestors in the distant past the skills of hunting and self-defense. In fact, the oldest known defensive objects are common cobblestones found in a cave in Ukraine. These round stones, which came from a nearby river, were supposedly used by the region's primitive inhabitants to defend themselves from potential predators. Pitching a projectile is a significant task for the delicate configuration of a humerus that barely articulates with the shoulder blade, which in turn only articulates at a very small joint with the clavicle, which itself articulates with the sternum, again by way of a very small joint. The entire stability of the shoulder depends on the muscles that move and support it.

The shoulder's wide range of movements is a great evolutionary advance, but it is also a source of problems. At times, the joint can move excessively, inducing luxation of the humerus head or damage to the soft tissues, among them, the brachial plexus. In fact, both upper and lower extremities are made by extension and fusion of the given somites. As muscles are made from more than one somite, nerves have to anastomose between them to allow a proper innervation of each muscle. This creates the necessity for a well-formed nerve plexus at the root of the limb.

The combination of a nerve plexus with a wide range of movement in a highly mobile joint at the shoulder creates the perfect scenario for a brachial plexus injury. In normal childbirth, there is already stretching of the brachial plexus as the infant's head and shoulder (usually the right one) are moved in opposite directions. Such injuries are always a possibility when the newborn is large and the mother's pelvis outlet is perhaps small; this is particularly true if the quality of obstetric attention is suboptimal.

As we grow, we start to move in multiple ways. Motorbikes and bicycles are economical transportation, particularly in big cities. They are relatively inexpensive, can adapt to small roads or to heavy traffic conditions and can be parked almost anywhere. But unfortunately, accidents are common. The head is perhaps protected with a helmet, but the shoulder remains exposed and can be separated violently from the head, inducing a great variety of brachial plexus injuries.

Once a brachial plexus injury is established, there exists a large array of treatment strategies. Conservative measures can help in some cases, but many injuries may need some sort of surgical repair. In these cases, nerve transfers opened a door allowing the repair of lesions once considered irrecoverable. In fact, even when a successful nerve suture, with or without intervening grafts was achieved, regenerating axons reached the distal muscles that were fibrotic and functionally dead. There is still much room for improvement: this is the arena of nerve root avulsions, particularly when all or almost all the brachial plexus nerve roots are avulsed. Some attempts to reimplant avulsed roots have been tried, but clinical results in humans have been dismal.

This book offers a new look at the field of brachial plexus injuries, taking advantage of the vast experience and knowledge of great figures who treated these dreadful conditions over many years. We hope the reader enjoys the book as much as the authors did writing it.

Vicente Vanaclocha
Assistant Professor
Department of Neurosurgery
Hospital General Universitario
Valencia, Spain

Nieves Sáiz-Sapena
University of Valencia
Valencia, Spain

Section 1

Introduction

Chapter 1

Introductory Chapter: Brachial Plexus Injuries - Past, Present, and Future

Vicente Vanaclocha and Nieves Saiz-Sapena

Additional information is available at the end of the chapter

http://dx.doi.org/10.5772/intechopen.81675

1. Introduction

Although they have a low incidence [1–3], brachial plexus injuries continue to be a cause of serious disability [4]. Their victims are mostly young people in the middle of their lives or newborns, always with worrisome long-term consequences [2–4]. Unfortunately brachial plexus lesions can also be the result of iatrogenic injuries [5]. The quality of life of those affected is devastated, with high personal [4, 6], familial [7], and societal costs [8, 9].

Nowadays, road accidents in young people continue to be the most common cause, particularly when the victim is thrown in the air and lands on the shoulder [2, 5, 10]. This is particularly common in developing Third World countries, where people have to recourse to the motorcycle for their daily transportation [1, 11–14], as a car is an option outside their reach. Other causes are wars [15–17] and assaults [18, 19]. The incidence is higher in males than in females [1, 2, 13, 20], probably related to the highest aggressiveness and violent behavior in the former [21]. In newborns brachial plexus injuries are usually due to problems during vaginal delivery [3, 22], particularly in case of a macrosomic fetus [23, 24], common in diabetic mothers [25]. In the developed countries, the fear of unpleasant medicolegal consequences in case of an obstetric brachial plexus injury has induced a significant increase in the proportion of cesarean section deliveries [26, 27]. The incidence of iatrogenic brachial plexus lesions unfortunately continues to be stable overtime with no signs of reduction [5, 28–30]. These iatrogenic lesions are induced while performing lymph node biopsy [5, 31, 32], vessel catheterization [33, 34], on applying radiotherapy in the treatment of cancer [35, 36] repairing upper limb bone fractures [37, 38], in programmed orthopedic procedures [39, 40], due to inadequate patient positioning [41, 42] or when restraining aggressive patients [43]. Preventing these iatrogenic injuries is particularly important, not only because they might lead to ugly medicolegal consequences [28] but because of our motto "primum non nocere" (first do no harm) [44]. Any measure or technical improvement aiming to decrease the chance of these unwanted iatrogenic injuries will always be most welcomed. Knowledge, awareness, and training of all hospital personnel must be a priority in our daily basis [45].

2. Treatment modalities

The age of the patient, the mechanism of injury (blunt or penetrating), the location (proximal or distal in the upper limb), and the extent of the lesion will influence the type and timing of the treatment algorithm as well as the final result [46, 47]. When all brachial plexus roots are affected, particularly if avulsed, there will be very limited treatment options, and the end results will be a severe upper limb disability with a very limited chance of a useful functional recovery [48–50].

Particularly, it is important to find out if the lesion is pre- or postganglionic as the first one has no chance of spontaneous recovery [51]. Magnetic resonance imaging has proven very useful in this respect [52]. Waiting for spontaneous recovery will entail an inexcusable waste of time that will lead to an unsatisfactory recovery [50, 53]. Thus, once the diagnosis of the nerve root avulsion is confirmed, the repair will have to be done as soon as the patient is able to tolerate the surgical procedure needed to be done [54, 55]. The "urgent" repair, a few days after injury, has been reported by some in cases of confirmed avulsion and in clean nerve sections (i.e., glass) [56].

The treatment strategy is based on the mechanism of injury [54], the findings of the physical and neurological examinations [57], and the results of the complementary diagnostic tests (electrodiagnostic studies [58], magnetic resonance imaging [59], and ultrasonography [60]). This last one is relatively inexpensive and can be made available to places with very limited resources [61]. It can also been used intraoperatively to see the anatomy of the damaged nerves, helping to decide if the lesioned nerve segment has to be removed and the gap grafted or a neurolysis will solve the problem [62]. The evolution of their results overtime is particularly useful to locate the lesion(s), assess its severity, and control the response to the treatments (physiotherapy, observation, surgical repair, electrostimulation, etc.) [63]. Computerized myelo-tomography was used in the past to diagnose the nerve root avulsions, but nowadays it has been replaced by magnetic resonance imaging [59, 64–66].

Spontaneous recovery can be expected in most brachial plexus injuries [67], particularly in the case of obstetric patients [68]. Among them the rate of spontaneous recovery is particularly high (66–92%) [69]. Physical therapy is essential to correct muscle contractures and avoid neglect of the damaged limb while waiting for spontaneous recovery [69]. In the case of inadequate recovery, on-time surgical treatment might be indicated [3, 68].

Progressive improvement of the surgical techniques with direct nerve repair, nerve grafting, and particularly with nerve transfers has greatly improved the results in the brachial plexus injuries [47, 70–72]. Direct repair, when at all possible, is still the first choice, provided that there is no tension in the suture line [73]. Nerve grafts are required to cover the gaps, but the results are often not as good as expected [74, 75]. Meanwhile, the nerve transfers have expanded our treatment capabilities with excellent results [72, 76]. They are particularly useful in nerve injuries affecting the distal parts of the upper limb, as other techniques like the nerve repair, direct or with nerve grafts, yield poor results [47, 70, 77]. The growing axons coming through the nerve repair take so long to reach the hand intrinsic muscles that when they do it find them atrophied and fibrotic [78–81]. Meanwhile, the nerve transfers provide new axons close to the injured muscles with an early and efficient repair [72, 76]. At times an end-to-side nerve transfer can be added to keep the muscles viable, while the growing axons from the direct primary nerve repair to reach their final destination in the motor end plates [82]. Nerve transfers solve the problem of a long distance between the lesion site and the motor end plates to be reinnervated [6, 49, 72, 76]. They can also be used in case of delayed patient referral [83] or dense scar at the primary injury site [84]. Sensory nerve transfer is another very promising area [85, 86], particularly in tetraplegic patients [87, 88], and can also help to control the neuropathic pain [89].

3. Future treatment possibilities

Currently, there is an intense research on pharmacological agents that accelerate the axonal regeneration, shortening the time needed to achieve the reinnervation [90, 91]. Other areas of research are the use of stem cells and growth factors as well as the search for artificial conduits that could substitute the autologous nerve grafts [90, 92]. The most serious injuries, the nerve root avulsions, are still awaiting an effective solution. Reimplantation has been attempted but the results are dismal [50].

Treatment of a complete brachial plexus avulsion with its resultant flail arm poses still a serious challenge [49]. Even with contralateral C_7 nerve root transfer, only some primitive movements are regained with limited use in the daily life [93]. Some have recommended upper limb amputation in these unfortunate cases [94].

Tetraplegic [88] and stroke [95] patient treatments are an area of expansion, aiming to recover some functions in the upper limbs that can improve their quality of life [88, 96]. The rationale behind is to use nerve transfers to recover specific functions (like finger movement) in areas of irreversible spinal cord or motor strip damage [76, 97].

Some technical refinements have been described attempting to reduce the chance of iatrogenic injury in cases of anesthetic brachial plexus block [98, 99]. The use of ultrasonography can be of invaluable help [100]. Some recommendations on patient positioning have also been forwarded [44]. The long-term commitment of every hospital employee is essential to minimize these unwanted mishaps.

4. The future in your own hospital

A final word should be said on how to start, develop, and consolidate a new peripheral nerve unit. This can be a major endeavor that demands continued devotion and long-term commitment. Once you start in this field, first you have to be known and accepted in your own hospital and then in your community. Time and persistence are needed to get the confidence of the referring doctors as well as the respect of the public. A stepwise and cautious attitude is recommended. While good results not always are acknowledged by our colleagues, a bad case can ruin our reputation. Meanwhile, to get the needed equipment and personnel is something that needs continuous negotiation with the hospital administrators; fighting for resources is also demanded by many other members of your own hospital. But with long-term persistence and unrestricted commitment, one usually achieves the goals, as proven by the authors of one of our following chapters.

5. Conclusions

Brachial plexus injuries continue to pose serious treatment dilemmas. Although the proximal injuries have a reasonable good prognosis, the distal ones not always get a good functional recovery. There has been a big improvement over the years, but research is needed to further improve the functional results, particularly in pan-brachial plexus avulsions. To start a new peripheral nerve unit is an exciting endeavor that demands enthusiasm, long-term commitment, and daily persistence.

Author details

Vicente Vanaclocha[1*] and Nieves Saiz-Sapena[2]

*Address all correspondence to: vvanaclo@hotmail.com

1 Department of Neurosurgery, Hospital General Universitario de Valencia, Valencia, Spain

2 Department of Anaesthesiology and Pain Treatment, Hospital 9 de Octubre de Valencia, Valencia, Spain

References

[1] Faglioni W, Siqueira MG, Martins RS, Heise CO, Foroni L. The epidemiology of adult traumatic brachial plexus lesions in a large metropolis. Acta Neurochirurgica. 2014;**156**(5):1025-1028

[2] Kaiser R, Waldauf P, Ullas G, Krajcová A. Epidemiology, etiology, and types of severe adult brachial plexus injuries requiring surgical repair: Systematic review and meta-analysis. Neurosurgical Review. Jul 17 2018. DOI: 10.1007/s10143-018-1009-2. [Epub ahead of print]

[3] Wall LB, Mills JK, Leveno K, Jackson G, Wheeler LC, Oishi SN, et al. Incidence and prognosis of neonatal brachial plexus palsy with and without clavicle fractures. Obstetrics and Gynecology. 2014;**123**(6):1288-1293

[4] Rasulić L, Savić A, Živković B, Vitošević F, Mićović M, Baščarević V, et al. Outcome after brachial plexus injury surgery and impact on quality of life. Acta Neurochirurgica. 2017;**159**(7):1257-1264

[5] Dengler NF, Antoniadis G, Grolik B, Wirtz CR, König R, Pedro MT. Mechanisms, treatment, and patient outcome of Iatrogenic injury to the brachial plexus-A retrospective single-center study. World Neurosurgery. 2017;**107**:868-876

[6] Dolan RT, Butler JS, Murphy SM, Hynes D, Cronin KJ. Health-related quality of life and functional outcomes following nerve transfers for traumatic upper brachial plexus injuries. The Journal of Hand Surgery, European Volume. 2012;**37**(7):642-651

[7] Oskay D, Oksüz C, Akel S, Firat T, Leblebicioğlu G. Quality of life in mothers of children with obstetrical brachial plexus palsy. Pediatrics International: Official Journal of the Japan Pediatric Society. 2012;**54**(1):117-122

[8] Felici N, Zaami S, Ciancolini G, Marinelli E, Tagliente D, Cannatà C. Cost analysis of brachial plexus injuries: Variability of compensation by insurance companies before and after surgery. Handchir Mikrochir Plast Chir Organ Deutschsprachigen Arbeitsgemeinschaft Handchir Organ Deutschsprachigen Arbeitsgemeinschaft Mikrochir Peripher Nerven Gefasse Organ V. 2014;**46**(2):85-89

[9] Pandey N, Gupta D, Mahapatra A, Harshvardhan R. Bed wise cost analysis of in-patient treatment of brachial plexus injury at a Level I trauma Center in India. Asian Journal of Neurosurgery. 2014;**9**(2):89-92

[10] Soldado F, Ghizoni MF, Bertelli J. Thoracodorsal nerve transfer for triceps reinnervation in partial brachial plexus injuries. Microsurgery. 2016;**36**(3):191-197

[11] Babar SM. Peripheral nerve injuries in a Third World country. The Central African Journal of Medicine. 1993;**39**(6):120-125

[12] Barman A, Chatterjee A, Prakash H, Viswanathan A, Tharion G, Thomas R. Traumatic brachial plexus injury: Electrodiagnostic findings from 111 patients in a tertiary care hospital in India. Injury. 2012;**43**(11):1943-1948

[13] Saadat S, Eslami V, Rahimi-Movaghar V. The incidence of peripheral nerve injury in trauma patients in Iran. Ulus Travma Ve Acil Cerrahi Derg Turk J Trauma Emerg Surg TJTES. 2011;**17**(6):539-544

[14] Suleiman FA, Almaaitah AA, Aqrabawi HE. Upper limb birth trauma in a Jordanian population: A prospective study at King Hussein Medical Centre, Amman, Jordan. JPMA: Journal of the Pakistan Medical Association. 2016;**66**(11):1422-1426

[15] Gousheh J. The treatment of war injuries of the brachial plexus. Journal of Hand Surgery. 1995;**20**(3 Pt 2):S68-S76

[16] Razaq S, Yasmeen R, Butt AW, Akhtar N, Mansoor SN. The pattern of peripheral nerve injuries among Pakistani soldiers in the war against terror. Journal of the College of Physicians and Surgeons--Pakistan. 2015;**25**(5):363-366

[17] Chambers JA, Hiles CL, Keene BP. Brachial plexus injury management in military casualties: Who, what, when, why, and how. Military Medicine. 2014;**179**(6):640-644

[18] Kibadi K, Portaels F, Pichot Y, Kapinga M, Moutet F. Stab wounds of the hand and forearm due to Kuluna in Kinshasa (Democratic Republic of Congo): Types of injuries and treatment. Revue Médicale de Bruxelles. 2015;**36**(6):468-474

[19] Bowles AO, Graves DE, Chiou-Tan FY. Distribution and extent of involvement in brachial plexopathies caused by gunshot wounds, motor vehicle crashes, and other etiologies: A 10-year electromyography study. Archives of Physical Medicine and Rehabilitation. 2004;**85**(10):1708-1710

[20] Valent F, Eleopra R, Manganotti P, Passadore P. A population-based study of injuries to the brachial plexus and to the peripheral nerves of the shoulder girdle and upper limb in the Italian region Friuli Venezia Giulia. Neurosurgical Review. 2018;**41**(2):519-523

[21] Stephenson Z, Woodhams J, Cooke C. Sex differences in predictors of violent and non-violent juvenile offending. Aggressive Behavior. 2014;**40**(2):165-177

[22] Grossman JAI, Price A, Chim H. Complications in surgery for brachial plexus birth injury: Avoidance and treatment. Journal of Hand Surgery. 2018;**43**(2):164-172

[23] Ouzounian JG. Risk factors for neonatal brachial plexus palsy. Seminars in Perinatology. 2014;**38**(4):219-221

[24] Okby R, Sheiner E. Risk factors for neonatal brachial plexus paralysis. Archives of Gynecology and Obstetrics. 2012;**286**(2):333-336

[25] Kc K, Shakya S, Zhang H. Gestational diabetes mellitus and macrosomia: A literature review. Annals of Nutrition & Metabolism. 2015;**66**(Suppl 2):14-20

[26] Gonen R, Bader D, Ajami M. Effects of a policy of elective cesarean delivery in cases of suspected fetal macrosomia on the incidence of brachial plexus injury and the rate of cesarean delivery. American Journal of Obstetrics and Gynecology. 2000;**183**(5):1296-1300

[27] Zuarez-Easton S, Shalev E, Salim R. Trend in major neonatal and maternal morbidities accompanying the rise in the cesarean delivery rate. Scientific Reports. 2015;**5**:12565

[28] Moore AE, Zhang J, Stringer MD. Iatrogenic nerve injury in a national no-fault compensation scheme: An observational cohort study. International Journal of Clinical Practice. 2012;**66**(4):409-416

[29] Po BT, Hansen HR. Iatrogenic brachial plexus injury: A survey of the literature and of pertinent cases. Anesthesia and Analgesia. 1969;**48**(6):915-922

[30] Huang Y. Iatrogenic injuries of the peripheral nerves: Analysis of 226 cases. Zhonghua Yi Xue Za Zhi. 1992;**72**(5):273-276, 318-316

[31] Davidson T, Malani A, Jones A. Brachial plexus traction injury following axillary node dissection. Clinical Oncology journal | The Royal College of Radiologists. 2000;**12**(6):419

[32] Ferencsik M, Piukovics K, Borbényi Z, Varga G. Peripheral nerve injuries as a rare complication of cervical lymph node excision for diagnostic purposes. Orvosi Hetilap. 1990;**131**(27):1465-1467

[33] Tong Z, Gu Y, Guo L, Guo J, Gao X, Li J, et al. An analysis of complications of brachial and axillary artery punctures. The American Surgeon. 2016;**82**(12):1250-1256

[34] Mulligan B, Espinosa GA, Mafee M. Prevention of brachial plexus injury during transaxillary artery catheterization. Military Medicine. 1983;**148**(6):518-520

[35] Gu B, Yang Z, Huang S, Xiao S, Zhang B, Yang L, et al. Radiation-induced brachial plexus injury after radiotherapy for nasopharyngeal carcinoma. Japanese Journal of Clinical Oncology. 2014;**44**(8):736-742

[36] Chen AM, Wang P-C, Daly ME, Cui J, Hall WH, Vijayakumar S, et al. Dose--volume modeling of brachial plexus-associated neuropathy after radiation therapy for head-and-neck cancer: Findings from a prospective screening protocol. International Journal of Radiation Oncology, Biology, Physics. 2014;**88**(4):771-777

[37] Khademolhosseini M, Abd Rashid AH, Ibrahim S. Nerve injuries in supracondylar fractures of the humerus in children: Is nerve exploration indicated? Journal of Pediatric Orthopaedics Part B. 2013;**22**(2):123-126

[38] Joiner ERA, Skaggs DL, Arkader A, Andras LM, Lightdale-Miric NR, Pace JL, et al. Iatrogenic nerve injuries in the treatment of supracondylar humerus fractures: Are we really just missing nerve injuries on preoperative examination? Journal of Pediatric Orthopedics. 2014;**34**(4):388-392

[39] Scully WF, Wilson DJ, Parada SA, Arrington ED. Iatrogenic nerve injuries in shoulder surgery. The Journal of the American Academy of Orthopaedic Surgeons. 2013; **21**(12):717-726

[40] Carofino BC, Brogan DM, Kircher MF, Elhassan BT, Spinner RJ, Bishop AT, et al. Iatrogenic nerve injuries during shoulder surgery. The Journal of Bone and Joint Surgery. American Volume. 2013;**95**(18):1667-1674

[41] Shimizu S, Sato K, Mabuchi I, Utsuki S, Oka H, Kan S, et al. Brachial plexopathy due to massive swelling of the neck associated with craniotomy in the park bench position. Surgical Neurology. 2009;**71**(4):504-508-509

[42] Desai KR, Nemcek AA. Iatrogenic brachial plexopathy due to improper positioning during radiofrequency ablation. Seminars in Interventional Radiology. 2011;**28**(2):167-170

[43] Guedes-Corrêa JF, Pereira MR da C, Torrão-Junior FJL, Martins JV, Barbosa DAN. A neglected cause of iatrogenic brachial plexus injuries in psychiatric patients. Neurosurgery. Mar 1, 2018;**82**(3):307-311. DOI: 10.1093/neuros/nyx162

[44] Duffy BJ, Tubog TD. The prevention and recognition of ulnar nerve and brachial plexus injuries. Journal of Perianesthesia Nursing: Official Journal of the American Society of PeriAnesthesia Nurses. 2017;**32**(6):636-649

[45] Blonna D, Wolf JM, Fitzsimmons JS, O'Driscoll SW. Prevention of nerve injury during arthroscopic capsulectomy of the elbow utilizing a safety-driven strategy. The Journal of Bone and Joint Surgery. American Volume. 2013;**95**(15):1373-1381

[46] Mohammad-Reda A. Early post-operative results after repair of traumatic brachial plexus palsy. Turkish Neurosurgery. 2013;**23**(1):1-9

[47] Ali ZS, Heuer GG, Faught RWF, Kaneriya SH, Sheikh UA, Syed IS, et al. Upper brachial plexus injury in adults: Comparative effectiveness of different repair techniques. Journal of Neurosurgery. 2015;**122**(1):195-201

[48] Abou-Al-Shaar H, Karsy M, Ravindra V, Joyce E, Mahan MA. Acute repair of traumatic pan-brachial plexus injury: Technical considerations and approaches. Neurosurgical Focus. 2018;**44**(Video Suppl 1):V4

[49] Liu Y, Lao J, Gao K, Gu Y, Zhao X. Functional outcome of nerve transfers for traumatic global brachial plexus avulsion. Injury. 2013;**44**(5):655-660

[50] Kachramanoglou C, Carlstedt T, Koltzenburg M, Choi D. Long-term outcome of brachial plexus reimplantation after complete brachial plexus avulsion injury. World Neurosurgery. 2017;**103**:28-36

[51] Limthongthang R, Bachoura A, Songcharoen P, Osterman AL. Adult brachial plexus injury: Evaluation and management. The Orthopedic Clinics of North America. 2013;**44**(4):591-603

[52] Karalija A, Novikova LN, Orädd G, Wiberg M, Novikov LN. Differentiation of pre- and postganglionic nerve injury using MRI of the spinal cord. PLoS One. 2016;**11**(12):e0168807

[53] Bertelli JA, Ghizoni MF. Reconstruction of C5 and C6 brachial plexus avulsion injury by multiple nerve transfers: Spinal accessory to suprascapular, ulnar fascicles to biceps branch, and triceps long or lateral head branch to axillary nerve. Journal of Hand Surgery. 2004;**29**(1):131-139

[54] Sinha S, Khani M, Mansoori N, Midha R. Adult brachial plexus injuries: Surgical strategies and approaches. Neurology India. 2016;**64**(2):289-296

[55] Gao K-M, Hu J-J, Lao J, Zhao X. Evaluation of nerve transfer options for treating total brachial plexus avulsion injury: A retrospective study of 73 participants. Neural Regeneration Research. 2018;**13**(3):470-476

[56] Pondaag W, van Driest FY, Groen JL, Malessy MJA. Early nerve repair in traumatic brachial plexus injuries in adults: Treatment algorithm and first experiences. Journal of Neurosurgery. 2018:1-7

[57] Thatte MR, Babhulkar S, Hiremath A. Brachial plexus injury in adults: Diagnosis and surgical treatment strategies. Annals of Indian Academy of Neurology. 2013;**16**(1):26-33

[58] Wiertel-Krawczuk A, Huber J. Standard neurophysiological studies and motor evoked potentials in evaluation of traumatic brachial plexus injuries—A brief review of the literature. Neurologia i Neurochirurgia Polska. Sep–Oct 2018;**52**(5):549-554. DOI: 10.1016/j.pjnns.2018.05.004

[59] Veronesi BA, Rodrigues MB, Sambuy MTCD, Macedo RS, Cho ÁB, Rezende MRD. Use of magnetic resonance imaging to diagnose brachial plexus injuries. Acta Ortopédica Brasileira. 2018;**26**(2):131-134

[60] Zhu Y-S, Mu N-N, Zheng M-J, Zhang Y-C, Feng H, Cong R, et al. High-resolution ultrasonography for the diagnosis of brachial plexus root lesions. Ultrasound in Medicine & Biology. 2014;**40**(7):1420-1426

[61] Chin B, Ramji M, Farrokhyar F, Bain JR. Efficient imaging: Examining the value of ultrasound in the diagnosis of traumatic adult brachial plexus injuries. A systematic review. Neurosurgery. Sep 1 2018;**83**(3):323-332. DOI: 10.1093/neuros/nyx483

[62] Burks SS, Cajigas I, Jose J, Levi AD. Intraoperative imaging in traumatic peripheral nerve lesions: Correlating histologic cross-sections with high-resolution ultrasound. Operative Neurosurgery (Hagerstown, Md.). 2017;**13**(2):196-203

[63] Marquez Neto OR, Leite MS, Freitas T, Mendelovitz P, Villela EA, Kessler IM. The role of magnetic resonance imaging in the evaluation of peripheral nerves following traumatic lesion: Where do we stand? Acta Neurochirurgica. 2017;**159**(2):281-290

[64] Fuzari HKB, Dornelas de Andrade A, Vilar CF, Sayão LB, Diniz PRB, Souza FH, et al. Diagnostic accuracy of magnetic resonance imaging in post-traumatic brachial plexus injuries: A systematic review. Clinical Neurology and Neurosurgery. 2017;**164**:5-10

[65] Martín Noguerol T, Barousse R, Socolovsky M, Luna A. Quantitative magnetic resonance (MR) neurography for evaluation of peripheral nerves and plexus injuries. Quantitative Imaging in Medicine and Surgery. 2017;**7**(4):398-421

[66] Wade RG, Itte V, Rankine JJ, Ridgway JP, Bourke G. The diagnostic accuracy of 1.5T magnetic resonance imaging for detecting root avulsions in traumatic adult brachial plexus injuries. The Journal of Hand Surgery, European Volume. Mar 2018;**43**(3):250-258. DOI: 10.1177/1753193417729587

[67] Lim SH, Lee JS, Kim YH, Kim TW, Kwon KM. Spontaneous recovery of non-operated traumatic brachial plexus injury. European Journal of Trauma and Emergency Surgery: Official Publication of the European Society for Trauma and Emergency Surgery. 2018;**44**(3):443-449

[68] Abid A. Brachial plexus birth palsy: Management during the first year of life. Orthopaedics & Traumatology: Surgery & Research. 2016;**102**(1 Suppl):S125-S132

[69] Raducha JE, Cohen B, Blood T, Katarincic J. A Review of Brachial Plexus Birth Palsy: Injury and Rehabilitation. Rhode Island Medical Journal (2013). 2017;**100**(11):17-21

[70] Hu C-H, Chang TN-J, Lu JC-Y, Laurence VG, Chuang DC-C. Comparison of Surgical strategies between proximal nerve graft and/or nerve transfer and distal nerve transfer based on functional restoration of elbow flexion: A retrospective review of 147 patients. Plastic and Reconstructive Surgery. 2018;**141**(1):68e-79e

[71] Wali AR, Santiago-Dieppa DR, Brown JM, Mandeville R. Nerve transfer versus muscle transfer to restore elbow flexion after pan-brachial plexus injury: A cost-effectiveness analysis. Neurosurgical Focus. 2017;**43**(1):E4

[72] Ray WZ, Chang J, Hawasli A, Wilson TJ, Yang L. Motor nerve transfers: A comprehensive review. Neurosurgery. 2016;**78**(1):1-26

[73] Bahm J, Gkotsi A, Bouslama S, El-Kazzi W, Schuind F. Direct nerve sutures in (extended) upper obstetric brachial plexus repair. Journal of Brachial Plexus and Peripheral Nerve Injury. 2017;**12**(1):e17-e20

[74] Haninec P, Sámal F, Tomás R, Houstava L, Dubovwý P. Direct repair (nerve grafting), neurotization, and end-to-side neurorrhaphy in the treatment of brachial plexus injury. Journal of Neurosurgery. 2007;**106**(3):391-399

[75] O'Grady KM, Power HA, Olson JL, Morhart MJ, Harrop AR, Watt MJ, et al. Comparing the efficacy of triple nerve transfers with nerve graft reconstruction in upper trunk obstetric brachial plexus injury. Plastic and Reconstructive Surgery. 2017;**140**(4):747-756

[76] Forli A, Bouyer M, Aribert M, Curvale C, Delord M, Corcella D, et al. Upper limb nerve transfers: A review. Hand Surgery & Rehabilitation. 2017;**36**(3):151-172

[77] Plate JF, Ely LK, Pulley BR, Smith BP, Li Z. Combined proximal nerve graft and distal nerve transfer for a posterior cord brachial plexus injury. Journal of Neurosurgery. 2013;**118**(1):155-159

[78] Wang ML, Rivlin M, Graham JG, Beredjiklian PK. Peripheral nerve injury, scarring, and recovery. Connective Tissue Research. Sep 6 2018:1-7. DOI: 10.1080/03008207.2018.1489381

[79] Kobayashi J, Mackinnon SE, Watanabe O, Ball DJ, Gu XM, Hunter DA, et al. The effect of duration of muscle denervation on functional recovery in the rat model. Muscle & Nerve. 1997;**20**(7):858-866

[80] Aydin MA, Mackinnon SE, Gu XM, Kobayashi J, Kuzon WM. Force deficits in skeletal muscle after delayed reinnervation. Plastic and Reconstructive Surgery. 2004; **113**(6):1712-1718

[81] Bertelli JA, Ghizoni MF. Nerve root grafting and distal nerve transfers for C5-C6 brachial plexus injuries. Journal of Hand Surgery. 2010;**35**(5):769-775

[82] Liao W-C, Chen J-R, Wang Y-J, Tseng G-F. The efficacy of end-to-end and end-to-side nerve repair (neurorrhaphy) in the rat brachial plexus. Journal of Anatomy. 2009; **215**(5):506-521

[83] Dy CJ, Baty J, Saeed MJ, Olsen MA, Osei DA. A population-based analysis of time to surgery and travel distances for brachial plexus surgery. Journal of Hand Surgery. 2016;**41**(9):903-909.e3

[84] Bahm J, El Kazzi W, Schuind F. Nerve transfers. Revue Médicale de Bruxelles. 2011;**32** (6 Suppl):S54-S57

[85] Bedeschi P, Celli L, Balli A. Transfer of sensory nerves in hand surgery. Journal of Hand Surgery (Edinburgh, Scotland). 1984;**9**(1):46-49

[86] Bertelli JA. Distal sensory nerve transfers in lower-type injuries of the brachial plexus. Journal of Hand Surgery. 2012;**37**(6):1194-1199

[87] Bertelli JA, Ghizoni MF, Tacca CP. Transfer of the teres minor motor branch for triceps reinnervation in tetraplegia. Journal of Neurosurgery. 2011;**114**(5):1457-1460

[88] Brown JM. Nerve transfers in tetraplegia I: Background and technique. Surgical Neurology International. 2011;**2**:121

[89] Emamhadi M, Andalib S. Nerve transfer to relieve pain in upper brachial plexus injuries: Does it work? Clinical Neurology and Neurosurgery. 2017;**163**:67-70

[90] Panagopoulos GN, Megaloikonomos PD, Mavrogenis AF. The present and future for peripheral nerve regeneration. Orthopedics. 2017;**40**(1, 1):e141-e156

[91] García Medrano B, Barrio Sanz P, Simón Pérez C, León Andrino A, Garrosa García M, Martín Ferrero MA, et al. Regeneration of critical injuries of the peripheral nerve with growth factors. Revista Española de Cirugía Ortopédica y Traumatología. 2013;**57**(3):162-169

[92] Rasulic L. Current concept in adult peripheral nerve and brachial plexus surgery. Journal of Brachial Plexus and Peripheral Nerve Injury. 2017;**12**(1):e7-e14

[93] Zhang C-G, Gu Y-D. Contralateral C7 nerve transfer–Our experiences over past 25 years. Journal of Brachial Plexus and Peripheral Nerve Injury. 2011;**6**(1):10

[94] Siqueira MG, Martins RS, Heise CO, Foroni L. Elective amputation of the upper limb is an option in the treatment of traumatic injuries of the brachial plexus? Arquivos de Neuro-Psiquiatria. 2017;**75**(9):667-670

[95] Zheng M-X, Hua X-Y, Feng J-T, Li T, Lu Y-C, Shen Y-D, et al. Trial of contralateral seventh cervical nerve transfer for spastic arm paralysis. The New England Journal of Medicine. 2018;**378**(1):22-34

[96] Senjaya F, Midha R. Nerve transfer strategies for spinal cord injury. World Neurosurgery. 2013;**80**(6):e319-e326

[97] Bryden AM, Peljovich AE, Hoyen HA, Nemunaitis G, Kilgore KL, Keith MW. Surgical restoration of arm and hand function in people with tetraplegia. Topics in Spinal Cord Injury Rehabilitation. 2012;**18**(1):43-49

[98] Jung MJ, Byun HY, Lee CH, Moon SW, Oh M-K, Shin H. Medial antebrachial cutaneous nerve injury after brachial plexus block: Two case reports. Annals of Rehabilitation Medicine. 2013;**37**(6):913-918

[99] Brull R, Hadzic A, Reina MA, Barrington MJ. Pathophysiology and etiology of nerve injury following peripheral nerve blockade. Regional Anesthesia and Pain Medicine. 2015;**40**(5):479-490

[100] Luftig J, Mantuani D, Herring AA, Nagdev A. Ultrasound-guided retroclavicular approach infraclavicular brachial plexus block for upper extremity emergency procedures. The American Journal of Emergency Medicine. 2017;**35**(5):773-777

Section 2

Biological Basis of Brachial Plexus Repair

Chapter 2

Tension in Peripheral Nerve Suture

Jörg Bahm, Tobias Esser, Bernd Sellhaus,
Wissam El-kazzi and Frederic Schuind

Additional information is available at the end of the chapter

http://dx.doi.org/10.5772/intechopen.78722

Abstract

Avoiding suture tension in peripheral nerve coaptation seems to be a clinical dogma since 30 years, although experimental data are weak and clinical practice shows good functional outcome after peripheral nerve repair by direct coaptation under "reasonable" tension, defined by *local anatomic feasibility* and the use of *specific suture material*. In this article, we focus on the microsurgical technique of nerve stump coaptation and the *distribution of tension through epineural sutures* with various suture materials; we also analyze the impact on the different nerve tissue layers, the limit of this approach and its combination with other tissue releasing techniques like *paraneurolysis, adjacent joint flexion, or bone shortening*.

Keywords: nerve suture, coaptation, tension, brachial plexus injury, obstetrical, peripheral nerve, microsurgery

1. Introduction

The actual state-of-the-art in suture-coaptation bringing together two stumps of a severed peripheral nerve requires good histologic quality of both stumps, a gap that may overcome by acceptable tension, and a good microsurgical technique when performing epineural or epi-perineural mattress sutures, leading finally to a nearly invisible congruent "anastomosis".

Few authors have dealt so far with aspects of technical improvement of nerve stump coaptation, but fascicular alignment seems to be a major factor to ensure proper regeneration [1].

Peripheral nerves contain elastic fibers and after nerve transsection, even without any loss of substance, a gap between the two stumps becomes apparent. The local nerve tissue damage and ingrowing fibrosis of both stumps may increase and/or fix the gap in an irreversible manner, than the further coaptation becomes hazardous.

Although "reasonable" tension may be applied to try to overcome the gap, it is generally recommended to perform nerve sutures in a tension-free environment using 9/0 and 10/0 microsurgical suture material. When these stitches break, a nerve graft is recommended.

Recently, we gained reasonable experience in the reconstruction of upper and extended upper obstetric brachial plexus lesions (OBPL) in general [2] and with direct sutures [3], showing very good clinical results of motor recovery after severe obstetric traction injury with complete trunk ruptures. Optimizing the functional result after surgical reconstruction in all types of OBPL is always the prevalent aim, especially to recover an adequate hand function [4].

The OBPL direct suture repair technique was introduced already over hundred years ago [5] and we know that several peripheral nerve surgeons are incline to perform a direct coaptation of two peripheral nerve stumps with a "reasonable" tension, to avoid short grafting with less dense nerve fiber interposition.

There is thus a striking controversy between a clinical axioma (tensionless nerve coaptation) and surgical experience, leading us to investigate this issue further and to discuss both the existing literature and possible research protocols.

2. Surgical technique

The nerve suture should bring together two stumps of good tissue quality, that is, free of fibrosis (i.e., infiltration of collagen fibers) or neuroma (predominance of misoriented peripheral minifascicles), with good fascicular appearance and a gap overcome by slight traction and finally hold by the sutures [6, 7]. de Medinaceli introduced a microsurgical technique focusing on good fascicular alignment in both stumps [1], mainly to avoid random fascicular ingrowth of the regeneration cones.

Every nerve microsurgeon knows that if there is tension, the first suture point is the most difficult to be achieved and at risk for filament rupture (**Figure 1**).

As there are more points added, the tension lowers (**Figure 2**) and at the end, the coaptation site shows a good appearance and mechanical resistance.

To prevent undue tension, either the proximal and/or the distal nerve stump may be mobilized, that is, freed from their paraneural tissue, thus giving additional length, gained at the price of decreased local blood supply (as the vasa nervorum might be interrupted by this circumferential paraneurolysis).

Also may one take advantage of the existence of "reserve capacity" of each peripheral nerve at the level of major joints, which are flexed to release more tissues.

In dramatic situations, like in war injuries or when considering very large nerve repairs (like the ischiatic nerve), bone shortening might be considered to reduce or overcome the gap.

http://dx.doi.org/10.5772/intechopen.78722

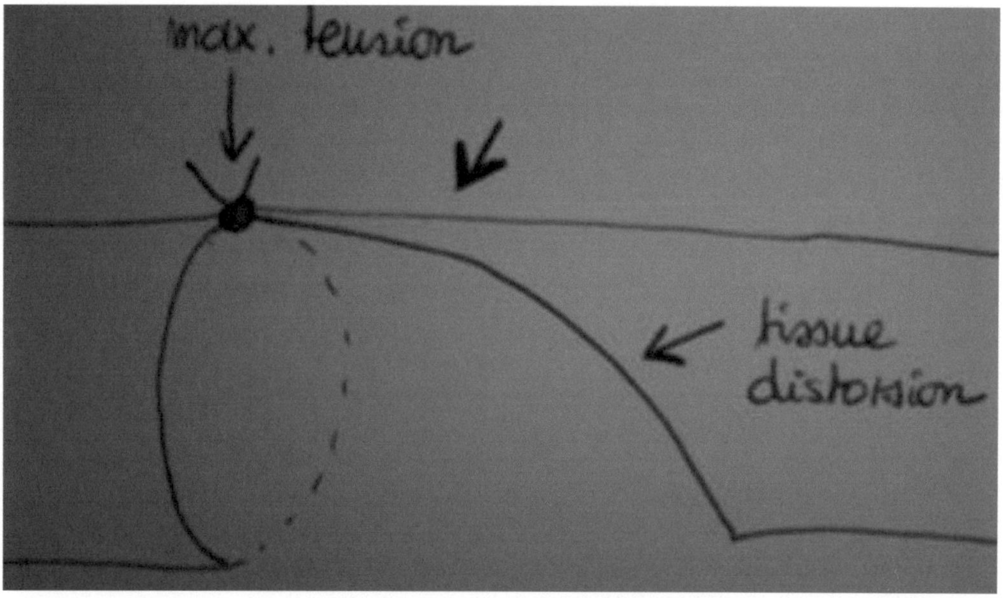

Figure 1. Problem of the first epineural suture knot under undue tension.

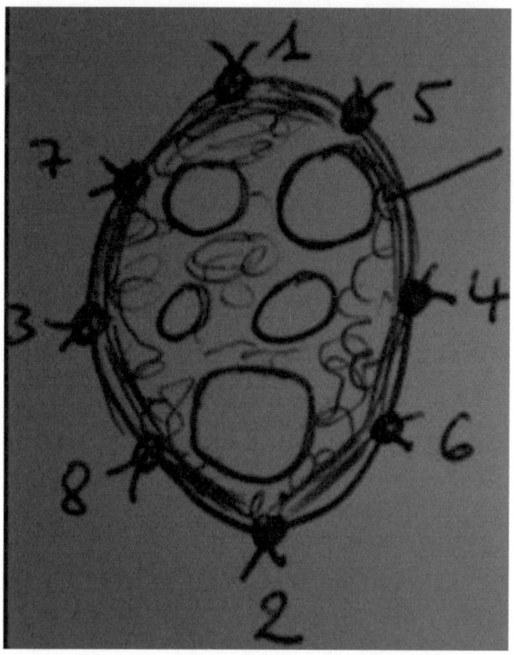

Figure 2. Tension decreases with more anchor points.

In very young children, like those suffering from OBPL, the structural elasticity of the longitudinally growing nerves is assumed to be enhanced, as is also the capacity of nerve regeneration and overall cortical plasticity. The young connective tissue is loose, nerve fibers and myelin sheaths are thin and the peripheral nerve structure itself is continually under a longitudinal growth stretch.

Concerning nerve stump coaptation at every age, there is no way to overcome the fascicular malalignment due to the intrinsic plexual structure constitutional of most multifascicular peripheral nerves (**Figure 3**).

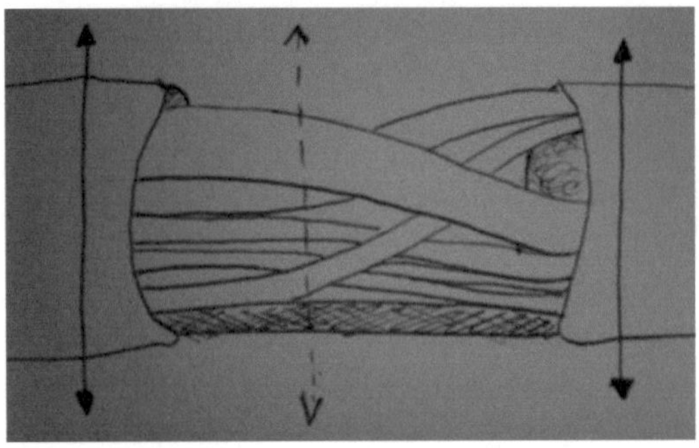

Figure 3. Intraneural plexiform fascicular structure.

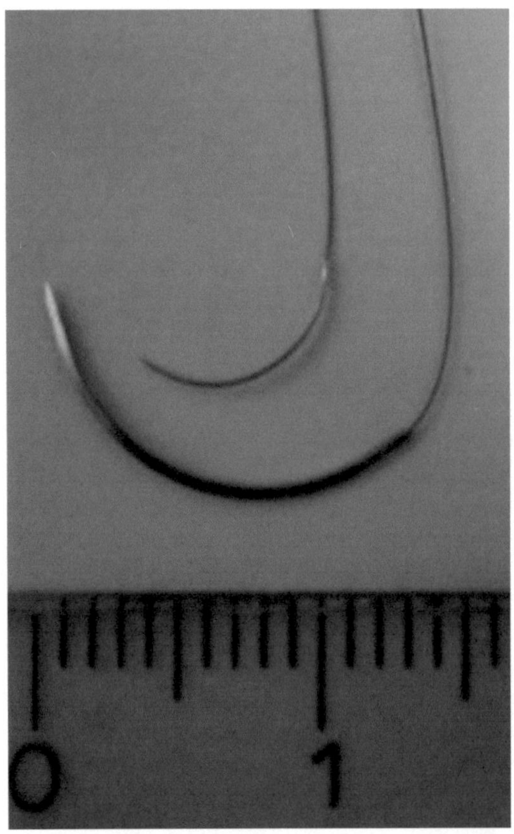

Figure 4. Onalon 6/0 microsurgical filament: fine needle, 6/0 strand.

http://dx.doi.org/10.5772/intechopen.78722

Moreover, we actually do not have an insight into the physiologic regeneration once the suture is completed and the wound is closed, as the diffusion tensor imaging (DTI) technology related to MRI images is actually not performed regularly after peripheral nerve surgery.

When it comes to the suture material, nerve microsurgeons routinely use 8–10 or 11/0 nylon (nonabsorbable monofilament) material with fine needles proportional to the filament diameter, that is, needles for 11/0 sutures are smaller and thinner than those for 8/0 sutures.

Recently, we developed in cooperation with Onatec (Pößneck Jestetten, Germany), a specific microsurgical suture material, made up of a 6/0 filament with a real microsurgical needle (**Figure 4**), allowing epineural nerve sutures of "bigger" nerves like the upper or middle trunk in OBPL repair or adult radial and median nerve coaptations.

As the 6/0 filament is inserted strictly epineural and thus lays outside the fascicular structures, and as nylon is supposed to be biologically inert, we continued that practice on a prospective series of OBPL repairs we actually published with a follow up of 18 months and still very promising results of sensory and motor function recovery [3].

Figures 5–7 show one clinical example of a typical upper and middle trunk neuroma repair with the identification of the rupture site (**Figure 5**), trimming of both proximal and distal stumps (**Figure 6**), and the direct suture (**Figure 7**).

The 6/0 strand together with a rather thick epineurium in larger nerves (like those mentioned above) gave us satisfactory coaptation stability already after two or three sutures, where

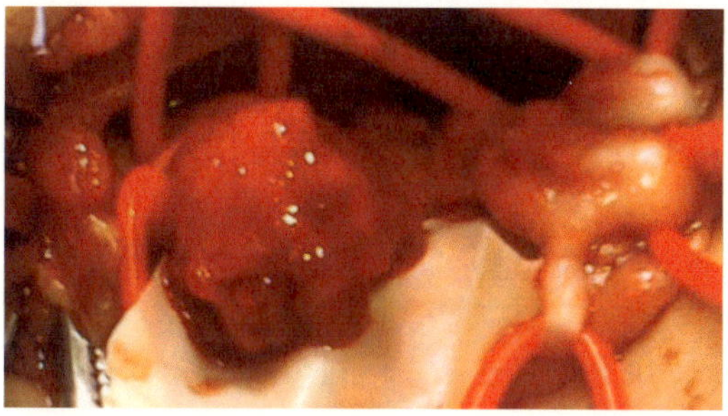

Figure 5. Clinical example of OBPL direct suture: upper and middle trunk rupture.

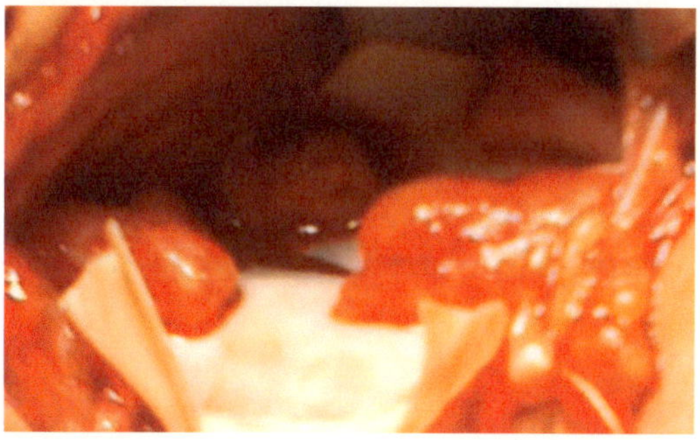

Figure 6. Clinical example of OBPL direct suture: after proximal and distal stump trimming.

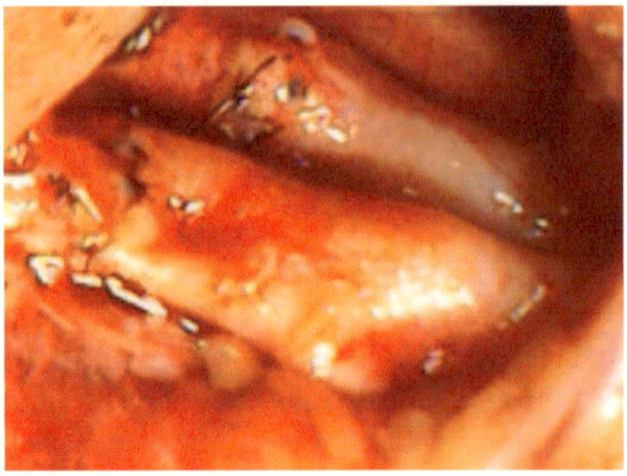

Figure 7. Clinical example of OBPL direct suture: upper and middle trunk direct suture.

thinner suture filaments needed more sutures to stabilize the coaptation. Nevertheless, in our OBPL trunk coaptations, we regularly used a minimum of 6–8 6/0 epineural sutures (**Figure 2**) before surrounding the coaptation site with a sleeve of fibrin glue.

The only similar stabilizing technique using foreign material promoted polylacton (vicryl) strips applied outside the epineurium to decrease the tension onto the suture points [8].

3. Morphologic and mechanic analysis

Tension is a force applied onto a surface and might be reduced on a circumference while using more anchor points (remind **Figure 2**). Suture tension has so far not been quantified or measured, we probably could state that it is even unmeasurable in the *in vivo* situation of a surgical procedure.

The question is how much of the maintained tension into the nerve stump coaptation is transmitted to the periphery, that is, the stumps, and if this affects nerve regeneration and the physiologic function afterwards.

Some experiences support the concept of a negative influence of nerve stretching on the physiologic function [9]. But clinical results show the feasibility of this method without lowering the functional outcome, even providing unexpected good results.

Tension could harm by decreasing the blood flow in the vasa nervorum (a stretch on a circular blood vessel-tube would flatten it and diminish the cross section, thus theoretically lower the blood flow); but one could argue that through the initial nerve lesion and the surgical paraneurolysis, those freed segments are anyhow separated from the local blood supply.

Tension is also said to increase local fibrosis (the amount of collagen fibers), but we should further investigate if the tension in the epineural layer, holding the suture material, is equally transmitted to the deeper structures (the deep interfascicular epineurium and finally the perineurium and the fascicular sheets).

http://dx.doi.org/10.5772/intechopen.78722

• Very young patient
• Acceptable nerve diameter (OBPL trunk or cord)
• Limited scar and/or gap
• Compliance for postoperative immobilization

Table 1. Ideal conditions for a direct suture approach.

• Good clinical result in OBPL direct sutures
• Longitudinal growth in young patients
• Tissue adaptation: elastic fibers, low collagen content, and postoperative immobilization

Table 2. Strong arguments for a limited tension-suture model.

One could imagine that the tension is hold within the thicker epineural layer of a thicker peripheral nerve and that the aligned fascicles in the nerve depth are no longer experiencing distraction stress—thus the nerve regeneration happening on the highways of the deeper fascicules would not be disturbed (that's what our clinical cases seem to show, like a "*tube-in-tube*" concept).

Tension is not measured easily, or even not at all, and once it comes to textbook descriptions like "reasonable tension" or "avoiding excessive tension" we should be convinced that the actually accepted dogma is weak.

On the other hand, there is the real danger of "promoting" bad microsurgical technique and overindication for direct coaptation, bringing together bad quality stumps under undue tension just to avoid a graft (donor site morbidity, longer procedure, two coaptation sites, but overall less fiber density).

Table 1 summarizes ideal clinical conditions for a direct suture approach; **Table 2** summarizes strong arguments for a limited tension, suture approach.

4. Literature research

Between 1975 and 2017, a PubMed MEDLINE research about "nerve suture" and "tension" only prompted eight valuable articles on nerve-suture related tension [8, 10–16]; presenting animal studies in rats, cats, dogs, and monkeys; using sciatic or upper limb nerves, and studying the outcome by histology and nerve conduction studies. There are so far no conclusive data about what is better and how much tension is tolerated.

5. Further investigations and today's conclusions

There is still enough controversy about tension tolerance in peripheral nerve surgery.

Clinical outcomes oppose to the experimental background, which on deeper analysis is rather weak, as the literature on the subject is scarce.

Out of our actual clinical and scientific knowledge, we believe that further investigation could be conducted in several ways:

- biomechanical analysis of various suture filament strengths used in nerve coaptation
- nylon suture: long term interaction with the fascicular anatomy studied by late histologic examination
- a model of a tube, in tube, behavior of the peripheral nerve (epineural versus fascicular tubes)
- in vivo observation of coapted nerves in a regeneration chamber.

Meanwhile, we continue to use all available "tricks" and refinements to decrease the gap and the suture tension, to allow optimal nerve fiber regeneration, without any visual help to follow this biological process after reconstructive surgery.

Never should our analysis allow bad techniques with insufficiently cleared stumps, undue tension on the coaptation after three or four knots, the introduction of stronger filament material (3 or 4/0), not adapted to the local anatomy, extension of the proposed technique to smaller nerves with fine epineurium, and not supporting suture material thicker than 10 or 11/0.

But with further developments, we may define indications and good surgical background conditions with limited nerve damage, good mobilization capacity of stumps, good microsurgical coaptation, and rewarded after a good technique with a significant functional result.

Author details

Jörg Bahm[1,3]*, Tobias Esser[1], Bernd Sellhaus[2], Wissam El-kazzi[3] and Frederic Schuind[3]

*Address all correspondence to: jorg.bahm@belgacom.net

1 Euregio Reconstructive Microsurgery Unit, Franziskus hospital Aachen, Germany

2 Institute for Neuropathology, RWTH University Hospital Aachen, Germany

3 Department for Orthopaedics and Traumatology, ULB Erasme University Hospital, Brussels, Belgium

References

[1] de Medinaceli L, Seaber AV. Experimental nerve reconnection: Importance of initial repair. Microsurgery. 1989;**10**:56-70

[2] Bahm J, Ocampo-Pavez C, Noaman H. Microsurgical technique in obstetric brachial plexus repair: A personal experience in 200 cases over 10 years. Journal of Brachial Plexus and Peripheral Nerve Injury. 2007;**2**:1

[3] Bahm J, Gkotsi A, Bouslama S, El-kazzi W, Schuind F. Direct nerve sutures in [extended] upper obstetric brachial plexus repair. Journal of Brachial Plexus and Peripheral Nerve Injury. 2017;**12**(1):e17-e20

[4] Kirjavainen M, Remes V, Peltonen J, Rautakorpi S, Helenius I, Nietosvaara Y. The function of the hand after operations for obstetric injuries to the brachial plexus. Journal of Bone and Joint Surgery (British). 2008;**90**(3):349-355

[5] Kennedy R. Suture of the brachial plexus in birth paralysis of the upper extremity. British Medical Journal. 1903;**1**(2197):298-301

[6] Millesi H. The nerve gap: Theory and clinical practice. Hand Clinics. 1986;**2**:651-663

[7] Trumble T. Overcoming defects in peripheral nerves. In: Gelberman RH, editor. Operative Nerve Repair and Reconstruction. Philadelphia: Lippincott; 1991

[8] Haas HG, Holste J. Spannungsentlastung bei Nähten peripherer Nerven. Handchirurgie, Mikrochirurgie, Plastische Chirurgie. 1990;**22**:156-162

[9] Driscoll PJ, Glasby MA, Lawson GM. An in vivo study of peripheral nerves in continuity: Biomechanical and physiological responses to elongation. Journal of Orthopaedic Research. 2002;**20**:370-375

[10] Hentz VR, Rosen JM, Xiao SJ, McGill KC, Abraham G. The nerve gap dilemma: A comparison of nerves repaired end to end under tension with nerve grafts in a primate model. Journal of Hand Surgery. 1993;**18**(3):417-425

[11] Maeda T, Hori S, Sasaki S, Maruo S. Effects of tension at the site of coaptation on recovery of sciatic nerve function after neurorrhaphy: Evaluation by walking-track measurement, electrophysiology, histomorphometry, and electron probe X-ray microanalysis. Microsurgery. 1999;**19**:200-207

[12] Miyamoto Y. Experimental study of results of nerve suture under tension vs. nerve grafting. Plastic and Reconstructive Surgery. 1979;**64**(4):540-549

[13] Okamoto H, Oka Y. Experimental study on tension and stretching to peripheral nerve. Nihon Seikeigeka Gakkai Zasshi. 1990;**64**(5):472-484

[14] Rodkey WG, Cabaud HE, McCarroll HR Jr. Neurorrhaphy after loss of a nerve segment: Comparison of epineurial suture under tension versus multiple nerve grafts. Journal of Hand Surgery. 1980;**5**(4):366-371

[15] Scherman P, Kanje M, Dahlin LB. Bridging short nerve defects by direct repair under tension, nerve grafts or longitudinal sutures. Restorative Neurology and Neuroscience. 2004;**22**(2):65-72

[16] Terzis J, Faibisoff B, Williams HB. The nerve gap: suture under tension vs. graft. Plastic and Reconstructive Surgery. 1975;**56**(2):166-170

Chapter 3

Plasticity in the Brain after a Traumatic Brachial Plexus Injury in Adults

Fernanda F. Torres, Bia L. Ramalho,
Cristiane B. Patroclo, Lidiane Souza,
Fernanda Guimaraes, José Vicente Martins,
Maria Luíza Rangel and Claudia D. Vargas

Additional information is available at the end of the chapter

http://dx.doi.org/10.5772/intechopen.77133

Abstract

In this chapter, we aim to discuss the neurophysiological basis of the brain reorganization (also called plasticity) that associates with a traumatic brachial plexus injury (TBPI), as well as following the brachial plexus surgical reconstruction and its physical rehabilitation. We start by reviewing core aspects of plasticity following peripheral injuries such as amputation and TBPI as well as those associated with chronic pain conditions. Then, we present recent results collected by our team centered on physiological measurements of plasticity after TBPI. Finally, we discuss that an important limitation in the field is the lack of systematic measurement of TBPI clinical features. We finish by proposing possible future venues in the domain of brain plasticity following a TBPI.

Keywords: cortical plasticity, traumatic brachial plexus injury, peripheral lesions, sensorimotor cortex, rehabilitation

1. Introduction

For a long time, synaptic networks in the brain were thought to be defined at birth and throughout the first years of life, remaining unchanged thereafter. However, contemporary research has shown that changes in functional brain organization do occur throughout an individual's life: synapses and dendritic budding are formed and eliminated, their efficacy being modulated through a complex network of neuronal interactions (reviewed in [1, 2]).

The term "plasticity" refers to the capacity for such changes [3, 4] occurring in response to injury, learning, training, illness or therapy [5]. Plasticity has been since then considered as an intrinsic property of the human brain, fundamental for overcoming genetic constraints and adapting to environmental pressures, physiological changes and new experiences [6].

Brain plasticity that follows a peripheral nervous system injury has been extensively documented at molecular, synaptic and systemic levels both in animal models and in humans. These plastic changes are, however, still documented at a purely descriptive level, and the search for conceptual models that allow predicting the direction of these changes is becoming mandatory [7]. Moreover, from a clinical point of view, the demonstration that the plasticity phenomenon underlies robust functional gain is necessary [5]. Progress in this direction should guide the development of new therapeutic interventions. This chapter starts with a brief introduction on brain plasticity after peripheral lesions with a special case for brachial plexus injury. We shall then discuss the available evidence of functional recuperation after surgery and physical therapy. Finally, we will point on new directions toward a fresh approach to changes in the brain following a peripheral nerve injury.

2. Brain plasticity

2.1. Brain plasticity after a peripheral injury

It is now widely demonstrated that lesions on the periphery of the body are capable of promoting structural and functional modification in the sensory (S1) and motor (M1) primary cortices [8, 9]. In animal models, these changes have been shown to translate into the topographic rearrangement of the body representation [10–13]. In patients who suffered traumatic amputation of a limb, noninvasive studies using the transcranial magnetic stimulation (TMS) technique showed that reorganizations in M1 are characterized by an expansion of the motor representation of the stump toward that of the segment of the amputated limb and, more rarely, an expansion of the face toward the amputated hand [14, 15]. Similarly, the analysis of the somatosensory reorganization resulting from amputation evidenced an extension of the face-to-hand representation in the primary somatosensory cortex [16] and more rarely, from the shoulder toward the hand [17], and from the trunk toward the hand [18]. However, recent results in these patients [19, 20] have shed doubt on the existence of face-to-hand expansion, suggesting instead that the territory of the missing hand is little, if so, invaded by neighboring representations after an amputation. In fact, it is possible to retrieve from stump muscles an EMG activity related specifically to the voluntarily evoked phantom hand movements [21], suggesting that the hand motor commands are preserved in the brain (reviewed in [22]). Furthermore, hand transplantation is capable of reversing the amputation-induced reorganization, with the intrinsic muscles of the donor hand being represented in M1 of the patients who received the transplant [23]. Cortical reorganization of intrinsic hand muscles was also verified in patients with leprosy affected by ulnar and median nerve injury [24]. Taken together, these results suggest that the sensorimotor representations in the brain are highly Mutable, that the hand representation persists in the sensorimotor cortex after an amputation and finally, that the changes following a peripheral lesion are reversible.

The mechanisms that underlie the occurrence of these plastic dynamics in the brain after injury and surgical reconstruction in the periphery of the body are still largely unknown and thus under active investigation. Different explanations such as neuronal budding and the unmasking of previously existing synapses, kept functionally silent by inhibitory gabaergic cortical circuits, are not mutually exclusive and should be taken into consideration [25, 26]. It is also possible that part of the observed reorganization is arising from subcortical plasticity and not only by new cortical–cortical projections [27, 28]. Furthermore, depending on the type of deafferentation, the mechanisms involved in the reorganization of the cortex might be different and could occur simultaneously at different levels of the sensorimotor system [27, 28].

2.2. Brain plasticity and pain

The phantom limb is a well-described phenomenon relating brain plasticity and limb amputation. When a persistent limb sensation occurs in the form of pain, the phenomenon is described as phantom limb pain [29]. Phantom pain has been shown to correlate with the degree of cortical reorganization [30, 31]. Using functional MRI, Lotze et al. [32] found a displacement of the cortical representation of the lips in M1 and S1 toward the representation of the hand in amputees, with a positive correlation between the displacement degree and the intensity of phantom pain. Furthermore, the imagined movement of the phantom hand activated the neighboring face area in the patients with phantom limb pain but not in the pain-free amputees. These data suggest selective coactivation of the cortical hand and mouth areas in patients with phantom limb pain [32].

The idea that cortical reorganization plays an important role in the pathophysiology of pain and that pain would lead to cortical reorganization has been confronted by the proposition that the plasticity generated by the phantom pain results both from the maintenance of the local cortical representations of the amputated limb and the disturbance of the interregional connectivity in the primary sensorimotor cortex [33]. However, it is possible that both processes (reorganization and preservation of limb function) occur simultaneously. Furthermore, the impact of peripheral factors such as afferent stimuli from the residual limb might be considered as an additional component in the pathology of phantom pain [34]. Besides, different experimental contexts, different methods for evaluation of cortical reorganization, and the difficulty in considering the impacts of psychological effects of the lesion seem to play an important explanatory role when one considers the variety of results in this domain, thus calling for the need to continue exploring this phenomenon [34].

Functional reorganization was also detected in pain syndromes. Flor et al. [35] investigated S1 reorganization in patients with chronic low back pain and observed a shift of the cortical representation of the back, interpreted as an expansion of the back's representation into the foot and leg area. Furthermore, Apkarian et al. [36] demonstrated that cortical gray matter density decreases regionally in chronic back pain patients. Other studies have also reported similar brain morphological changes related to various chronic pain conditions such as complex regional pain syndrome [37], chronic headache [38], and fibromyalgia [39]. The Apkarian group, in a series of revisions, further proposes that the transition from acute to chronic pain would be due to learning mechanisms within the cortical–limbic circuitry, leading to the formation of continuously reinforced memories that could not be extinguished, as a consequence of motivational and emotional associations with the painful stimuli, possibly potentiated by a greater learning capacity due to a predisposition to addictive behavior [40].

2.3. A model for brain plasticity investigation: brachial plexus injury

The brachial plexus (PB) is composed of a set of peripheral nerves responsible for the sensory, motor and autonomic innervation of the upper limb. Injury to peripheral nerve structures and/or medullary avulsion as a result of a traumatic brachial plexus injury (TBPI) lead to changes in cortical representations [41–44] and are also often associated with neuropathic pain [45]. Surgical procedures have been used in the treatment of TBPI patients with a view to the partial reconstruction of the lost innervation [46]. In particular, the nerve transfer technique (neurotization) has been described as effective for restoring denervated muscle function, particularly in cases where spinal root avulsions are involved [47]. However, the complete reconstruction of the motor bundles that innervate the arm after a TBPI is still not possible and priorities have been established to guide reconstructive strategies, the rescue of elbow flexion being the main purpose of the more prevalent cirurgical procedures [48–50]. As an important cirurgical outcome, Htut et al. [51] showed that pain reduction was greater for the group of patients who underwent grafting and nerve transfer and that pain intensity was lower for the group of patients submitted to surgery than for those who did not undergo the procedure.

Mano et al. [41] and Malessy et al. [42] were pioneers in the study of cortical plasticity in patients with TBPI employing transcranial magnetic stimulation. Since then, a few studies have been published in order to evaluate these plastic phenomena. After surgical transfer of the intercostal to the musculocutaneous nerve, a shift from medial to lateral of the biceps representation in M1 cortical map was reported [41, 43]. However, after this surgical procedure the tactile stimulation of the newly innervated forelimb skin area often results in tactile sensation in the chest region [52–54]. The neurotization of the biceps with fibers from the contralateral C7 root is another possible strategy to rescue elbow flexion. C7 root fibers are normally involved in adduction and extension of the ipsilateral arm. With this neurotization, flexion of the injured arm will no longer be under the control of the contralateral hemisphere, but rather under the control of the ipsilateral hemisphere. The cerebral hemisphere ipsilateral to the injured plexus will be controlling both the extension of the intact arm and flexion of the neurotized arm. In a fMRI study, performing an elbow flexion after the contralateral C7 neurotization of the biceps resulted in a bilateral cortical activity in a network comprising the premotor and primary motor cortex as well as the posterior parietal and supplementary motor areas ipsilateral to the neurotized arm [44].

In a fMRI longitudinal study, Yoshikawa et al. [55] accompanied 20 TBPI patients before and up to 32 months after different TBPI surgeries. Patients were asked to perform or simulate flexion/extension elbow movements with the affected arm. A reduction in the elbow movements representation in the contralateral sensorimotor cortex was observed at approximately 3 months after injury, reducing further after 1 year of injury (9 months of surgery). Over time, as the functional recovery of the elbow movements occurred, a concurrent reemergence of the activation areas was observed in the sensorimotor cortex.

Employing resting state fMRI Fraiman et al. [56] analyzed the empirical functional correlations between neighboring voxels. They found evidence of faster correlation decay as a function of distance in the M1 region corresponding to the upper limb but not in the face area in patients with TBPI as compared to a control group. A possible mechanism to explain the lowered correlation between neighboring voxels as compared to control subjects would be due to reduced activity in the intrinsic horizontal network, which is thought to orchestrate motor synergies in M1. Interestingly, these modifications also encompassed the M1 trunk/lower limb representation, suggesting that TBPI might imply in a bodily extended motor dysfunction. Accordingly, it was also found that TBPI affects body balance [57]. Souza et al. [57] showed that TBPI patients oscillate more in the sagittal plane as compared to a control group while standing barefoot on a force platform for 60s.

Liu et al. [58] and Hsieh et al. [59] explored changes in interhemispheric functional connectivity, observing decreased connectivity and loss of cortical inhibition between the primary motor areas of the two hemispheres after TBPI. Fraiman et al. [56] also found faster correlation decay as a function of distance in ipsilateral M1. Lu et al. [60], using voxel-based morphometry in fMRI, found less gray matter in BPI patients in brain regions such as the cerebellum, the anterior cingulate cortex, the bilateral inferior, medial and superior frontal lobes and bilateral insula, most regions closely related to motor functions. The authors speculate that this loss of gray matter might be the neural basis for the difficulties in motor rehabilitation of BPI patients. Other studies have explored further aspects of cortical plasticity after TBPI. Employing resting-state fMRI, Feng et al. [61] investigated differences between right and left injuries in right handed individuals revealing that right limb injuries induce greater cortical reorganization. Moreover, plasticity does not seem to be restricted to the sensorimotor cortex, involving higher-order regions such as the precuneus, the lateral aspect of the posterior parietal cortex, the superior parietal lobe, and the intraparietal sulcus [62]. Taken together, these results call for a more careful evaluation of the functional loss after TBPI.

Socolovsky et al. [63] recently reviewed different factors that could play a role in neuroplasticity and functional regeneration after nerve transfer. Distance between cortical territories of the donor and receptor nerves, the presence of preexisting brain connections, gross versus fine movement restoration, rehabilitation, brain trauma and age at lesion were listed as influencing functional restoration [63].

Rangel [64] employed an action observation and electroencephalogram (EEG) paradigm to investigate if a TBPI affects the capacity to anticipate the occurrence of sensory and motor events in the space around the arm. If it was the case, a change in the neural signature specific to each context (observation of a hand movement or of a hand about to be touched by an external object) might be verified. Preliminary results showed that the electrophysiological marker associated to predicting actions was preserved in the left sensorimotor region when TBPI patients with incomplete lesions sparing the hand observed actions performed by a right hand. Crucially, the ability to estimate upcoming touch events in the hand was preserved only for the sensorimotor cortex contralateral to the spared limb, suggesting a dependency of online sensory information to estimate events around the hand.

2.4. Clinical impact of TBPI

Although cortical plasticity after TBPI and its reconstruction has already been widely demonstrated [41–44, 46, 55, 56, 58, 59, 61–63], it is still very challenging to evaluate its clinical impact. Below we speculate about some reasons for that fact.

The first reason is that TBPI outcomes are still underestimated. It is known that TBPI consequences go beyond motor disability and pain. It also includes psychic, social and quality of life impairment [65, 66]. Since TBPIs are complex and heterogeneous, it is not expected that a single measure should completely cover all these aspects [67]. However, TBPI outcome reports are routinely limited to motor function, specially muscle strength, most frequently measured through British Medical Research Council (BMRC or MRC) scale [68]. Notwithstanding, TBPI may lead to limitations in various daily living activities such as washing, dressing, combing, eating, and preparing meals, in addition to restricting social participation, such as work, hanging out with friends and practicing sports. All this can have a strong impact on the individual's lifestyle [69, 70]. A cohort study followed 629 polytraumatized patients to evaluate the influence of upper extremity trauma on in-hospital progress, rehabilitation and social situation in the long term. The subgroup with TBPI presented slightly worse scores on mental and physical components of the quality of life survey SF-12 and significantly worse results in the score used to classify the rehabilitation status, which included a self-assessment of individual, social, financial, professional and medical items and a questionnaire and examination performed by the surgeon. Furthermore, the average duration of rehabilitation was more than twice as long, there were significantly longer duration of unemployment and higher retraining rate for TBPI patients when compared to other injuries [71]. Besides, there is a gap regarding the assessment of activities and social participation post-TBPI [72]. In a recent systematic review, Hill et al. [69] found that upper limb activities are rarely evaluated for this population, and there is still a shortage of clinimetric evidence in the questionnaires used to assess activity after TBPI. As a consequence, the major cortical plasticity measures take only motor function and their brain-related changes as their outcomes. It is possible that nonmotor consequences of TBPI also result from cortical plasticity driven by mechanisms still unrecognized and unexplored. This knowledge may open new doors to access and understand cortical plasticity.

Another reason lies on the research protocols to evaluate cortical plasticity after a TBPI. Many factors that may also influence cortical plasticity are frequently disconsidered, for example: dominance [41, 43, 59], side of injury [58], cause of injury [55, 59, 61], associated traumas [41–44, 55], physical therapy treatment [42–44, 55, 56, 59, 61] and pain relief medication [41–44, 55, 56, 59, 61]. Several factors influence the execution of activities by the upper limb, besides hand dominance. Some activities require unimanual and others, bimanual skill [73]. Furthermore, individuals with TBPI can adapt to their injury over time, performing tasks with their unaffected limb, changing handedness or compensating by using other body parts [74]. In addition, it is known that tasks performed by the upper limbs are complex, requiring control of positioning and multiple joints in varying degrees of freedom [75, 76]. This situation prevents the translation of experimental evidence into useful tools in clinical practice.

2.5. TBPI rehabilitation impact on cortical plasticity

A better understanding of cortical plasticity in TBPI may improve patients outcomes through the development of more accurate prognostic measures and more effective and customized therapies. Surgical treatments such as nerve, muscle and tendon transfers require plasticity to have good results (reviewed in [63]); therefore, after surgical treatment, specific approaches should be performed according to the type of surgery to which the patient was submitted. For example, in neurotization or nerve transfer, physical therapy should involve muscles related to the donor's nerve [43, 77–79]. The patient initially performs movements of the target muscle through the activation of the donor nerve muscles and this synergism will be useful in the beginning of the treatment to gain strength at the target muscle. Recently, Dahlin et al. [79] reported a case of a TBPI patient, who was initially treated with a transfer of intercostal to musculocutaneous nerve. Due to insufficient recovery of elbow flexion, after 2 years, he received a gracilis muscle transfer reinnervated by a phrenic nerve transfer. Electromyographic measurement showed that different activation patterns of the biceps and gracilis muscles were evoked by coughing and deep breathing, respectively. Moreover, voluntary elbow flexion elicited activity in the biceps and gracilis muscles associated with a decreased activity in intercostal muscles. These results corroborate findings [41, 43] indicating that the neural control of elbow flexion in M1 gradually separates from the control of voluntary breathing. In addition, it brings important information for elaborating therapy protocols concerning which specific task would be encouraged in order to facilitate elbow flexion (i.e., transferring coughing function in patients operated with intercostal nerve transfer and transferring deep breathing function in case of phrenic nerve transfer).

Moreover, Souza et al. [57] showed that motor impairment after TBPI is not restricted to the upper limb segment, since the clinical balance assessment and posturographic analysis in a TBPI group indicate that these individuals do exhibit balance impairments. This study indicated that rehabilitation after TBPI should not be directed only to the upper limb, but also to prevent and treat the secondary outcomes of this condition.

The TBPI rehabilitation team, therefore, must have a good understanding of the cerebral changes caused by the injury, the surgical reconstruction and the physical therapy, so that an individually tailored rehabilitation program can be applied according to the injury characteristics and the functional problems experienced by the patient in order to guide plasticity so that the best possible clinical outcome can be achieved [79]. Many TBPI rehabilitation programs are purely empirical, but recent studies have suggested that specific interventions could accelerate axon regeneration and brain plasticity [80, 81]. There is accumulating evidence that central adaptation factors are relevant to the recovery following peripheral trauma, which may also contribute to optimal functional outcomes. The modulation of the central nervous system is a key component of current rehabilitation strategies, being it sensory re-education, constraint induced movement therapy, exercise, electrical stimulation or transcranial stimulation [82]. Further studies investigating brain plasticity following TBPI rehabilitation with a longitudinal design are needed to a better understanding of the natural history of the disease, the cerebral response to the injury and changes following rehabilitation through the potential approach of guided plasticity.

2.6. Relevance

Improving knowledge on TBPI and its treatment is also an opportunity to reduce its social and economic impacts, the main victims being in general male in working age. Since Narakas' report in 1985 [50], subsequent series on brachial plexus injury around the world reaffirmed the importance of motor vehicle accidents, especially motorcycle, as its main cause [83–89]. The same trend is observed in series covering peripheral nerve injury in general [90–93].

However, traffic accidents as a whole, including motorcycle ones, impact more intensely in developing countries [94]. As an example of this situation, in Brazil, a huge increase by 400% in motorcycle fleet was observed from 2003 to 2015 [95]. In recent years, there grew up from 20 million in 2012 to more than 25 million in 2017 [96]. A consequent increase in motorcycle accidents reports should be naturally expected. However, official data show that the relative contribution to traffic accidents by motorcycle is much higher than could be previously imagined. In the first 6 months of 2017, motorcycles represented 27% of total Brazilian vehicular fleet, but were responsible for 74% of total indemnity paid by traffic accidents in the same period. Since traffic accidents involving motorcycles represent the most frequent cause of TBPI [83–89], an increase in TBPI in the Brazil, and in other developing countries, can be predicted in the near future.

3. Conclusions

There is mounting evidence that the brain is capable of recognizing and incorporating new information after a peripheral lesion followed by its surgical reconstruction. Frequently, these plastic processes are associated with persisting pain, a phenomenon that has been shown to correlate with the degree of cortical reorganization. However, the mechanisms underlying these phenomena are still only partially uncovered. TBPI is an interesting model of brain plasticity due to its incidence, the large variety of injury levels and the available surgical reconstructive procedures. For instance, studies with TBPI have shown changes in cortical representation after surgical transfer. Shortcomings in interpreting the results from studies relating brain changes after TBPI and its reconstruction are the paucity of systematic correlation of TBPI with detailed clinical evaluation protocols and the need of further investigation of physical therapy outcomes after TBPI. New venues in this domain shall be opened through the development of approaches allowing putting together more detailed clinical investigation protocols and that of brain mechanisms associated to plasticity after TBPI.

Acknowledgements

This work is part of the ABRAÇO Initiative for the Brachial Plexus Injury (http://abraco.numec.prp.usp.br/) of the Fundação de Amparo à Pesquisa do Estado de São Paulo (FAPESP)'s Research, Innovation and Dissemination Center for Neuromathematics (grant 2013/07699-0, http://neuromat.numec.prp.usp.br/). It was also supported by the Conselho Nacional de Pesquisa (CNPq) (grants 306817/2014-4 and 309560/2017-9) and the Fundação de Amparo à Pesquisa do Rio de Janeiro FAPERJ (grants E-26/111.655/ 2012, E26/010.002902/2014 and E-26/010.002474/2016).

http://dx.doi.org/10.5772/intechopen.77133

Conflict of interest

The authors declare that there is no conflict of interest.

Author details

Fernanda F. Torres[1,2], Bia L. Ramalho[1,2], Cristiane B. Patroclo[1,2], Lidiane Souza[1,2], Fernanda Guimaraes[2,3], José Vicente Martins[2], Maria Luíza Rangel[1,2] and Claudia D. Vargas[1,2]*

*Address all correspondence to: claudiadvargas@gmail.com

1 Laboratory of Neurobiology of movement, Institute of Biophysics Carlos Chagas Filho, Federal University of Rio de Janeiro, Rio de Janeiro, Brazil

2 Laboratory of Neuroscience and Rehabilitation, Institute of Neurology Deolindo Couto, Federal University of Rio de Janeiro, Rio de Janeiro, Brazil

3 Federal Institute of Rio de Janeiro, Rio de Janeiro, Brazil

References

[1] Buonomano DV, Merzenich MM. Cortical plasticity: From synapses to maps. Annual Review of Neuroscience. 1998;**21**:149-186. DOI: 10.1146/annurev.neuro.21.1.149

[2] Nudo RJ. Adaptive plasticity in motor cortex: Implications for rehabilitation after brain injury. Journal of Rehabilitation Medicine. 2003;(41 Suppl):7-10. DOI: 10.1080/16501960310010070

[3] Merzenich MM, Kaas JH, Wall JT, Sur M, Nelson RJ, Felleman DJ. Progression of change following median nerve section in the cortical representation of the hand in areas 3b and 1 in adult owl and squirrel monkeys. Neuroscience. 1983;**10**(3):639-665. DOI: 10.1016/0306-4522(83)90208-7

[4] Kaas JH. Plasticity of sensory and motor maps in adult mammals. Annual Review of Neuroscience. 1991;**14**(1):137-167. DOI: 10.1146/annurev.ne.14.030191.001033

[5] Cramer SC, Sur M, Dobkin BH, O'Brien C, Sanger TD, Trojanowski JQ, et al. Harnessing neuroplasticity for clinical applications. Brain. 2011;**134**(Pt 6):1591-1609. DOI: 10.1093/brain/awr039

[6] Pascual-Leone A, Amedi A, Fregni F, Merabet LB. The plastic human brain cortex. Annual Review of Neuroscience. 2005;**28**:377-401. DOI: 10.1146/annurev.neuro.27.070203.144216

[7] Nudo RJ. Mechanisms for recovery of motor function following cortical damage. Current Opinion in Neurobiology. 2006;**16**(6):638-644. DOI: 10.1016/j.conb.2006.10.004

[8] Lundborg G. Nerve injury and repair – A challenge to the plastic brain. Journal of the Peripheral Nervous System. 2003;**8**:209-226. DOI: 10.1111/j.1085-9489.2003.03027.x

[9] Kaas JH, Florence SL. Reorganization of sensory and motor systems in adult mammals after injury. In: Kaas JH, editor. The Mutable Brain: Dynamic and Plastic Features of the Developing and Mature Brain. Amsterdam: Harwood Academic Publishers; 2001

[10] Merzenich MM, Kaas JH, Wall J, Nelson RJ, Sur M, Felleman D. Topographic reorganization of somatosensory cortical areas 3b and 1 in adult monkeys following restricted deafferentation. Neuroscience. 1983;**8**:33-55. DOI: 10.1016/0306-4522(83)90024-6

[11] Sanes JN, Suner S, Donoghue JP. Dynamic organization of primary motor cortex output to target muscles in adult rats. I. Long-term patterns of reorganization following motor or mixed peripheral nerve lesions. Experimental Brain Research. 1990;**79**:479-491. DOI: 10.1007/BF00229318

[12] Pons TP, Garraghty PE, Ommaya AK, Kaas JH, Taub E, Mishkin M. Massive cortical reorganization after sensory deafferentation in adult macaques. Science. 1991;**252**(5014):1857-1860. DOI: 10.1126/science.1843843

[13] Merzenich MM, Jenkins WM. Reorganization of cortical representations of the hand following alterations of skin inputs induced by nerve injury, Skin Island transfers, and experience. Journal of Hand Therapy. 1993;**6**(2):89-104. DOI: 10.1016/S0894-1130(12)80290-0

[14] Cohen LG, Bandinelli S, Findley TW, Hallett M. Motor reorganization after upper limb amputation in man. A study with focal magnetic stimulation. Brain. 1991;**114**(Pt 1B):615-627. DOI: 10.1093/brain/114.1.615

[15] Mercier C, Reilly KT, Vargas CD, Aballea A, Sirigu A. Mapping phantom movement representations in the motor cortex of amputees. Brain. 2006;**129**:2202-2210. DOI: 10.1093/brain/awl180

[16] Borsook D, Becerra L, Fishman S, Edwards A, Jennings CL, Stojanovic M, et al. Acute plasticity in the human somatosensory cortex following amputation. Neuroreport. 1998 Apr 20;**9**(6):1013-1017. DOI: 10.1097/00001756-199804200-00011

[17] Kew JJ, Halligan PW, Marshall JC, Passingham RE, Rothwell JC, Ridding MC, et al. Abnormal access of axial vibrotactile input to deafferented somatosensory cortex in human upper limb amputees. Journal of Neurophysiology. 1997;**77**:2753-2764. DOI: 10.1152/jn.1997.77.5.2753

[18] Knecht S, Henningsen H, Elbert T, Flor H, Höhling C, Pantev C, et al. Reorganizational and perceptional changes after amputation. Brain. 1996 Aug;**119**(Pt 4):1213-1219. DOI: 10.1093/brain/119.4.1213

[19] Makin TR, Scholz J, Henderson Slater D, Johansen-Berg H, Tracey I. Reassessing cortical reorganization in the primary sensorimotor cortex following arm amputation. Brain. 2015;**138**:2140-2146. DOI: 10.1093/brain/awv161

[20] Makin TR, Bensmaia SJ. Stability of sensory topographies in adult cortex. Trends in Cognitive Sciences. 2017;**21**:195-204. DOI: 10.1016/j.tics.2017.01.002

[21] Reilly KT, Mercier C, Schieber MH, Sirigu A. Persistent hand motor commands in the amputees' brain. Brain. 2006;**129**(Pt 8):2211-2223. DOI: 10.1093/brain/awl154

[22] Reilly KT, Sirigu A. The motor cortex and its role in phantom limb phenomena. The Neuroscientist. 2008 Apr;**14**(2):195-202. DOI: 10.1177/1073858407309466

[23] Vargas CD, Aballéa A, Rodrigues EC, Reilly KT, Mercier C, Petruzzo P, et al. Re-emergence of hand-muscle representations in human motor cortex after hand allograft. Proceedings of the National Academy of Sciences of the United States of America. 2009;**28**:7197-7202. DOI: 10.1073/pnas.0809614106

[24] Batista e Sá VW, Gomes MK, Rangel ML, Sanchez TA, Moreira FA, et al. Primary motor cortex representation of handgrip muscles in patients with leprosy. PLoS Neglected Tropical Diseases. 2015;**9**(7):e0003944. DOI: 10.1371/journal.pntd.0003944

[25] Rossini PM, Pauri F. Neuromagnetic integrated methods tracking human brain mech anisms of sensorimotor areas 'plastic' reorganisation. Brain Research Reviews. 2000;**33**: 131-154. DOI: 10.1016/S0169-328X(00)00090-5

[26] Jacobs K, Donoghue J. Reshaping the cortical motor map by unmasking latent intracortical connections. Science. 1991;**251**:944-947. DOI: 10.1126/science.2000496

[27] Kambi N, Halder P, Rajan R, Arora V, Chand P, Arora M, et al. Large-scale reorganization of the somatosensory cortex following spinal cord injuries is due to brainstem plasticity. Nature Communications. 2014;**5**:1-10. DOI: 10.1038/ncomms4602

[28] Garraghty PE, Kaas JH. Functional reorganization in adult monkey thalamus after peripheral nerve injury. Neuroreport. 1991;**2**(12):747-750. DOI: 10.1146/annurev.ne.14.030191.001033

[29] Melzack R. Phantom limbs and the concept of a neuromatrix. Trends in Neurosciences. 1990;**13**(3):88-92. DOI: 10.1016/0166-2236(90)90179-E

[30] Flor H, Elbert T, Knecht S, Wienbruch C, Pantev C, Birbaumer N, et al. Phantom-limb pain as a perceptual correlate of cortical reorganization following arm amputation. Nature. 1995;**375**(6531):482-484. DOI: 10.1038/375482a0

[31] Lotze M, Grodd W, Birbaumer N, Erb M, Huse E, Flor H. Does use of a myoelectric prosthesis prevent cortical reorganization and phantom limb pain? Nature Neuroscience. 1999;**2**(6):501-502. DOI: 10.1038/9145

[32] Lotze M, Flor H, Grodd W, Larbig W, Birbaumer N. Phantom movements and pain. An fMRI study in upper limb amputees. Brain. 2001;**124**(Pt 11):2268-2277. DOI: 10.1093/brain/124.11.2268

[33] Makin TR, Cramer AO, Scholz J, Hahamy A, Slater DH, Tracey I, et al. Deprivation-related and use-dependent plasticity go hand in hand. eLife. 2013;**2**:1-15. DOI: 10.7554/eLife.01273

[34] Andoh J, Milde C, Tsao JW, Flor H. Cortical plasticity as a basis of phantom limb pain: Fact or fiction? Neuroscience. 2017. DOI: 10.1016/j.neuroscience.2017.11.015

[35] Flor H, Knost B, Birbaumer N. Processing of pain- and body-related verbal material in chronic pain patients: Central and peripheral correlates. Pain. 1997;**73**(3):413-421. DOI: 10.1016/S0304-3959(97)00137-1

[36] Apkarian AV, Sosa Y, Sonty S, Levy RM, Harden RN, Parrish TB, et al. Chronic back pain is associated with decreased prefrontal and thalamic gray matter density. The Journal of Neuroscience. 2004;**24**(46):10410-10415. DOI: 10.1523/JNEUROSCI.2541-04.2004

[37] Maihöfner C, Handwerker HO, Neundörfer B, Birklein F. Patterns of cortical reorganization in complex regional pain syndrome. Neurology. 2003;**61**(12):1707-1715. DOI: 10.1212/01.WNL.0000098939.02752.8E

[38] Schmidt-Wilcke T, Leinisch E, Straube A, Kämpfe N, Draganski B, Diener HC, et al. Gray matter decrease in patients with chronic tension type headache. Neurology. 2005;**65**(9):1483-1486. DOI: 10.1212/01.wnl.0000183067.94400.80

[39] Kuchinad A, Schweinhardt P, Seminowicz DA, Wood PB, Chizh BA, Bushnell MC. Accelerated brain gray matter loss in fibromyalgia patients: Premature aging of the brain? The Journal of Neuroscience. 2007;**27**(15):4004-4007. DOI: 10.1523/JNEUROSCI.0098-07.2007

[40] Mansour AR, Farmer MA, Baliki MN, Apkarian AV. Chronic pain: The role of learning and brain plasticity. Restorative Neurology and Neuroscience. 2014;**32**(1):129-139. DOI: 10.3233/RNN-139003

[41] Mano Y, Nakamuro T, Tamura R, Takayanagi T, Kawanishi K, Tamai T, et al. Central motor reorganization after anastomosis of the Musculocutaneous and intercostal nerves following cervical root avulsion. Annals of Neurology. 1995;**38**:15-20. DOI: 10.1002/ana.410380106

[42] Malessy MJA, Wim K, Thomeer RTWM, Dijk JG. Cortical excitability of the biceps muscle after intercostal-to-Musculocutaneous nerve transfer. Neurosurgery. 1998;**42**:787-794. DOI: 10.1097/00006123-199804000-00062

[43] Malessy MJA, Bakker D, Dekker AJ, Vandijk G, Thomeer RTWM. Functional magnetic resonance imaging and control over the biceps muscle after intercostal–musculocutaneous nerve transfer. Journal of Neurosurgery. 2003;**98**:261-268. DOI: 10.3171/jns.2003.98.2.0261

[44] Beaulieu JY, Blustajn J, Teboul F, Baud P, Schonen S, Thiebaud JB, et al. Cerebral plasticity in crossed C7 grafts of the brachial plexus: An fMRI. Microsurgery. 2006;**26**:303-310. DOI: 10.1002/micr.20243

[45] Apkarian AV, Bushnell MC, Treede RD, Zubieta JK. Human brain mechanisms of pain perception and regulation in health and disease. European Journal of Pain. 2005;**9**:463-484. DOI: 10.1016/j.ejpain.2004.11.001

[46] Anastakis DJ, Malessy MJA, Chen R, Davis KD, Mikulis D. Cortical plasticity following nerve transfer in the upper extremity. Hand Clinics. 2008;**24**:425-444. DOI: 10.1016/j.hcl.2008.04.005

[47] Ray WZ, Mackinnon SE. Management of nerve gaps: Autografts, allografts, nerve transfers, and end-to-side neurorrhaphy. Experimental Neurology. 2010;**223**(1):77-85. DOI: 10.1016/j.expneurol.2009.03.031

[48] Millesi H. Surgical management of brachial plexus injuries. Journal of Hand Surgery. 1977;**2**:367-379. DOI: 10.1016/S0363-5023(77)80046-4

[49] Narakas A. Brachial plexus surgery. The Orthopedic Clinics of North America. 1981;**12**: 303-323

[50] Narakas A. The treatment of brachial plexus injuries. International Orthopaedics. 1985;**9**(1): 29-36. DOI: 10.1007/BF00267034

[51] Htut M, Misra P, Anand P, Birch R, Carlstedt T. Pain phenomena and sensory recovery following brachial plexus avulsion injury and surgical repairs. Journal of Hand Surgery (British). 2006;**31**:596-605. DOI: 10.1016/j.jhsb.2006.04.027

[52] Yeh CDC-C, M-C WF-C. Intercostal nerve transfer of the musculocutaneous nerve in avulsed brachial plexus injuries: Evaluation of 66 patients. The Journal of Hand Surgery. 1992;**17A**(5):822-828. DOI: 10.1016/0363-5023(92)90451-T

[53] Kawai H. Intercostal nerve transfer. In: Kawai H, Kawabata H, editors. Brachial Plexus Palsy. Singapura: World Scientific Publishing Co.; 2000. pp. 161-236

[54] Ramalho BL. Investigação da sensibilidade superficial e sensação referida em participantes com lesão e reconstrução cirúrgica do plexo braquial. Rio de Janeiro: Federal University of Rio de Janeiro; 2015 In Portuguese

[55] Yoshikawa T, Hayashi H, Tajiri Y, Satake Y, Ohtomo K. Brain reorganization in patients with brachial plexus injury: A longitudinal functional MRI study. The Scientific World Journal. 2012;**501751**:1-11. DOI: 10.1100/2012/501751

[56] Fraiman D, Miranda MF, Erthal F, Buur PF, Elschot M, Souza L, et al. Reduced functional connectivity within the primary motor cortex of patients with brachial plexus injury. NeuroImage Clinical. 2016;**12**:277-284. DOI: 10.1016/j.nicl.2016.07.008

[57] Souza L, Lemos T, Silva DC, de Oliveira JM, Guedes Correa JF, Tavares PL, et al. Balance impairments after brachial plexus injury as assessed through clinical and posturographic evaluation. Frontiers in Human Neuroscience. 2016;**9**:715. DOI: 10.3389/fnhum.2015.00715

[58] Liu B, Li T, Tang WJ, Zhang JH, Sun HP, Xu WD, et al. Changes of inter-hemispheric functional connectivity between motor cortices after brachial plexuses injury: A resting-state fMRI study. Neuroscience. 2013;**243**:33-39. DOI: 10.1016/j.neuroscience.2013.03.048

[59] Hsieh JC, Cheng H, Hsieh H-M, Liao K-K, Wu Y-T, Yeh T-C, et al. Loss of Interhemispheric inhibition on the Ipsilateral primary sensorimotor cortex in patients with brachial plexus injury: fMRI study. Annals of Neurology. 2002;**51**:381-385. DOI: 10.1002/ana.10149

[60] Lu Y, Liu H, Hua X, Xu JG, Gu YD, Shen Y. Attenuation of brain grey matter volume in brachial plexus injury patients. Neurological Sciences. 2016;**37**(1):52-56. DOI: 10.1007/s10072-015-2356-1

[61] Feng JT, Liu HQ, Xu JG, Gu YD, Shen YD. Differences in brain adaptive functional reorganization in right and left total brachial plexus injury patients. World Neurosurgery. 2015;**84**:702-708. DOI: 10.1016/j.wneu.2015.04.046

[62] Feng JT, Liu HQ, Hua XY, Gu YD, Xu JG, Xu WD. Brain functional network abnormality extends beyond the sensorimotor network in brachial plexus injury patients. Brain Imaging and Behavior. 2016;**10**(4):1198-1205. DOI: 10.1007/s11682-015-9484-3

[63] Socolovsky M, Malessy M, Lopez D, Guedes F, Flores L. Current concepts in plasticity and nerve transfers: Relationship between surgical techniques and outcomes. Neurosurgical Focus. 2017;**42**(3):E13. DOI: 10.3171/2016.12.FOCUS16431

[64] Rangel MLS. Predição de eventos ocorrendo no espaço ao redor da mão: um estudo eletroencefalográfico em indivíduos saudáveis e em pacientes com lesão de plexo braquial [thesis]. Rio de Janeiro: Universidade Federal do Rio de Janeiro; 2015 In Portuguese

[65] Mancuso CA, Lee SK, Dy CJ, Landers ZA, Model Z, Wolfe SW. Expectations and limitations due to brachial plexus injury: A qualitative study. Hand (New York, N. Y.). 2015;**10**(4):741-749. DOI: 10.1007/s11552-015-9761-z

[66] Franzblau L, Chung KC. Psychosocial outcomes and coping after complete avulsion traumatic brachial plexus injury. Disability and Rehabilitation. 2015;**37**(2):135-143. DOI: 10.3109/09638288.2014.911971

[67] Bengtson KA, Spinner RJ, Bishop AT, Kaufman KR, Coleman-Wood K, Kircher MF, et al. Measuring outcomes in adult brachial plexus reconstruction. Hand Clinics. 2008;**24**(4):401-415. DOI: 10.1016/j.hcl.2008.04.001

[68] Dy CJ, Garg R, Lee SK, Tow P, Mancuso CA, Wolfe SW. A systematic review of outcomes reporting for brachial plexus reconstruction. The Journal of Hand Surgery. 2015;**40**(2):308-313. DOI: 10.1016/j.jhsa.2014.10.033

[69] Hill BE, Williams G, Bialocerkowski AE. Clinimetric evaluation of questionnaires used to assess activity after traumatic brachial plexus injury in adults: A systematic review. Archives of Physical Medicine and Rehabilitation. 2011;**92**(12):2082-2089. DOI: 10.1016/j.apmr.2011.07.188

[70] Novak CB, von der Heyde RL. Evidence and techniques in rehabilitation following nerve injuries. Hand Clinics. 2013;**29**(3):383-392. DOI: 10.1016/j.hcl.2013.04.012

[71] Macke C, Winkelmann M, Mommsen P, Probst C, Zelle B, Krettek C, Zeckey C. Injuries to the upper extremities in polytrauma: Limited effect on outcome more than ten years after injury - a cohort study with 629 patients. The Bone & Joint Journal. 2017;**99B**(2):255-260. DOI: 10.1302/0301-620X.99B2.37999

[72] Hill BE, Dip G, Williams G, Olver J, Bialocerkowski AE. Do existing patient-report activity outcome measures accurately reflect day-to-day arm use following adult traumatic

brachial plexus injury? Journal of Rehabilitation Medicine. 2015;**47**(5):438-444. DOI: 10.2340/16501977-1950

[73] Kilbreath SL, Heard RC. Frequency of hand use in healthy older persons. The Australian Journal of Physiotherapy. 2005;**51**(2):119-122. DOI: 10.1016/S0004-9514(05)70040-4

[74] Eggers IM, Mennen U. The evaluation of function of the flail upper limb classification system: Its application to unilateral brachial plexus injuries. The Journal of Hand Surgery. 2001;**26**(1):68-76. DOI: 10.1053/jhsu.2001.20159

[75] van Meeteren J, van Rijn RM, Selles RW, Roebroeck ME, Stam HJ. Grip strength parameters and functional activities in young adults with unilateral cerebral palsy compared with healthy subjects. Journal of Rehabilitation Medicine. 2007;**39**(8):598-604. DOI: 10.2340/16501977-0095

[76] Michielsen ME, de Niet M, Ribbers GM, Stam HJ, Bussman JB. Evidence of a logarithmic relationship between motor capacity and actual performance in daily life of the paretic arm following stroke. Journal of Rehabilitation Medicine. 2009;**41**(5):327-331. DOI: 10.2340/16501977-0351

[77] Liu Y, Lao J, Gao K, Gu Y, Zhao X. Functional outcome of nerve transfers for traumatic global brachial plexus avulsion. Injury. 2013;**44**(5):655-660. DOI: 10.1016/j.injury.2012.02.006

[78] Chalidapong P, Sananpanich K, Klaphajone J. Electromyographic comparison of various exercises to improve elbow flexion following intercostal nerve transfer. Journal of Bone and Joint Surgery. British Volume (London). 2006;**88**(5):620-622. DOI: 10.1302/0301-620X.88B5.17360Chalidapong

[79] Dahlin LB, Andersson G, Backman C, Svensson H, Björkman A. Rehabilitation, using guided cerebral plasticity, of a brachial plexus injury treated with intercostal and phrenic nerve transfers. Frontiers in Neurology. 2017;**8**:72. DOI: 10.3389/fneur.2017.00072

[80] Duffau H. Brain plasticity: From pathophysiological mechanisms to therapeutic applications. Journal of Clinical Neuroscience. 2006;**13**(9):885-897. DOI: 10.1016/j.jocn.2005.11.045

[81] Gordon T, English AE. Strategies to promote peripheral nerve regeneration: Electrical stimulation and/or exercise. The European Journal of Neuroscience. 2016;**43**(3):336-350. DOI: 10.1111/ejn.13005

[82] Simon NG, Franz CK, Gupta N, Alden T, Kliot M. Central adaptation following brachial plexus injury. World Neurosurgery. 2015. DOI: 10.1016/j.wneu.2015.09.027

[83] Faglioni W Jr, Siqueira MG, Martins RS, Heise CO, Foroni L. The epidemiology of adult traumatic brachial plexus lesions in a large metropolis. Acta Neurochirurgica. 2014;**156**(5):1025-1028. DOI: 10.1007/s00701-013-1948-x

[84] Flores LP. Epidemiological study of the traumatic brachial plexus injuries in adults. Arquivos de Neuro-Psiquiatria. 2006;**64**(1):88-94. DOI: /S0004-282X2006000100018

[85] Mello Junior JS, Souza TCR, Andrade FG, Castaneda L, Baptista AF, Nunes K, et al. Perfil Epidemiológico de Pacientes com Lesão Traumática do Plexo Braquial avaliados em um Hospital Universitário no Rio de Janeiro, Brasil, 2011. Revista Brasileira de Neurologia. 2012;**48**(3):5-8

[86] Moraes FB, Kwae MY, Silva RP, Porto CC, Magalhães DP, Paulino MV. Aspectos clínicos de pacientes com lesão traumática do plexo braquial após tratamento cirúrgico. Revista Brasileira de Ortopedia. 2015;**50**(5):556-561. DOI: 10.1016/j.rbo.2015.04.006

[87] Dubuisson AS, Kline DG. Brachial plexus injury: A survey of 100 consecutive cases from a single service. Neurosurgery. 2002;**51**(3):673-682. DOI: 10.1227/01.NEU.0000023600.59365.41

[88] Midha R. Epidemiology of brachial plexus injuries in a multitrauma population. Neurosurgery. 1997;**40**(6):1182-1188. DOI: 10.1097/0006123-199706000-00014

[89] Kim DH, Murovic JA, Tiel RL, Kline DG. Mechanisms of injury in operative brachial plexus lesions. Neurosurgical Focus. 2004;**16**(5):E2

[90] Asplund M, Nilsson M, Jacobsson A, von Holst H. Incidence of traumatic peripheral nerve injuries and amputations in Sweden between 1998 and 2006. Neuroepidemiology. 2009;**32**(3):217-228. DOI: 10.1159/000197900

[91] Ciaramitaro P, Mondelli M, Logullo F, Grimaldi S, Battiston B, Sard A, et al. Italian network for traumatic neuropathies. Traumatic peripheral nerve injuries: Epidemiological findings, neuropathic pain and quality of life in 158 patients. Journal of the Peripheral Nervous System. 2010;**15**(2):120-127. DOI: 10.1111/j.1529-8027.2010.00260.x

[92] Eser F, Aktekin LA, Bodur H, Atan C. Etiological factors of traumatic peripheral nerve injuries. Neurology India. 2009;**57**(4):434-437. DOI: 10.4103/0028-3886.55614

[93] Kouyoumdjian JA. Peripheral nerve injuries: A retrospective survey of 456 cases. Muscle & Nerve. 2006;**34**(6):785-788. DOI: 10.1002/mus.20624

[94] Global Status Report on Road Safety 2015. Geneva: World Health Organization. p. 2015

[95] Seerig LM, Bacchieri G, Nascimento GG, Barros AJD, Demarco FF. Use of motorcycle in Brazil: Users profile, prevalence of use and traffic accidents occurrence — A population-based study. Ciênc. saúde coletiva. 2016;**21**(12):3703-3710. DOI: 10.1590/1413-812320152112.28212015.2016

[96] Seguradora Líder DPVAT. Boletim Estatístico - Ano 07. 2017;**2**

Section 3

Brachial Plexus Injury Repair

Chapter 4

Nerve Root Reimplantation in Brachial Plexus Injuries

Vicente Vanaclocha-Vanaclocha,
Nieves Saiz-Sapena, José María Ortiz-Criado and
Leyre Vanaclocha

Additional information is available at the end of the chapter

http://dx.doi.org/10.5772/intechopen.82431

Abstract

Nerve root avulsion is the most severe form of brachial or lumbosacral plexus injury. Spontaneous recovery is extremely rare, and when all the nerve roots of the affected plexus are avulsed, the therapeutic options are very limited. Nerve root reimplantation has been attempted since the 1990s, first in experimental animal models and afterwards in human beings. Currently, only partial recovery of the proximal limb muscles has been achieved. New therapeutic strategies have been developed to improve motor neuron survival and axonal regeneration, with promising results. Neurotrophic factors and some drugs have been used successfully to improve the regenerating ability, but long-term studies in humans are needed to develop complete recovery of the affected limb.

Keywords: brachial plexus injury, nerve root avulsion, nerve root reimplantation, motor neuron death, muscle atrophy, neurotrophic factor, axonal regeneration, motor and sensory recovery

1. Introduction

A common event in brachial plexus (BP) injury is nerve root avulsion (NRA) in which the nerve rootlets (NRts) are torn from the spinal cord (SC) [1–3]. Once avulsed, the NRts retract towards the nerve root (NR) sleeve [4]. The most common cause is traumatic NR stretching due to road accidents or parturitions [3, 5]. These injuries can also happen but are much rarer at the lumbosacral plexus [6]. The ventral rootlets (motor) are weaker and thus get injured more often and more seriously than their posterior counterparts [7].

Soon after avulsion anterior horn motor neurons (MN) and sensory neurons at the dorsal root ganglion (DRG) undergo apoptosis [8–17]. Inside the avulsed NR itself, there is a Wallerian degeneration with axonal and myelin loss [18]. The muscles, devoid of nervous impulses, undergo atrophy and fibrous transformation [19, 20]. At the SC, the neurons suffer loss of synapses with destruction of previous neuronal networks and creation of new anomalous ones that will lead to abnormal nerve impulses which might induce chronic neuropathic pain [21–24].

After complete NRA, spontaneous regeneration is impossible [9]. In case of a single NRA, recovery coming from nearby healthy ones can be expected in neonates but not in adult patients [25]. Ventral root surgical reimplantation has been attempted both in experimental animals and in human beings with partial recovery [26, 27].

Axonal regeneration is stronger in direct ventral NR reimplantation [26, 28]. This is rarely possible [4, 7, 29, 30], so peripheral nerve grafts (NGs) are used to cover the gap between the SC and the remains of the avulsed NR [31–33]. These NGs are usually taken from a peripheral sensory nerve (medial antebrachial cutaneous, radial cutaneous, and saphenous), which is not the ideal situation as motor nerve regeneration is worse if sensory nerves are used as donors compared to mixed or pure motor nerves [34–36]. Acellular conduits have also been used, but the regeneration does not grow further than 2 cm [37, 38].

1.1. Historical background

Surgical repair of spinal NRs after traumatic avulsion in live human beings was considered technically impossible until the pioneering work of Carlstedt et al. [39]. The first studies were done in rats [40], then in cats [41] and finally in primates [42, 43], before attempting NR reimplantation in humans [44]. Initially, the efforts were directed at repairing the ventral rootlets (motor), but in adult human beings, it provided only mild improvement in shoulder and elbow movements [45]. In children, some hand movement was recovered but with limited function [29]. In addition, it was found that the number of surviving MNs and the number of axons that regenerated after NR reimplantation had a direct relationship with the final functional recovery [7, 30]. Ever since, many research groups have focussed on understanding the underlying pathophysiology and to find surgical strategies and drugs that can enhance regenerating capacities.

2. Pathophysiology

The interface between the central and peripheral nervous systems is known as the transitional zone (TZ) [46], and the regenerating capacities are influenced by both of them. The first is rich in astrocytes that create channels through which motor fibers pass [15]. The latter has Schwann cells that secrete neurotrophic factors (NFs) with higher regeneration abilities [47].

NRA disconnects the transverse arch that exists at each spinal level between the posterior horn sensory, the lateral horn autonomic and anterior horn neurons [23] as well as disconnection of the DRG neurons from the bulbar and thalamic sensory nuclei [48]. NRA also induces loss of synapses and dendritic arborisation, fiber degeneration, neuronal death, posterior spinal column degeneration and glial proliferation [23, 48]. The synaptic and neuronal changes in the posterior horn produce neuropathic pain [24, 48, 49].

NRA is followed by an intense inflammatory SC reaction [50] with microglia, macrophage and glial proliferations [51]. At the TZ a dense scar tissue and a neuroma from the avulsed MN develop [15, 46, 52–55]. In the normal situation, the central nervous system is rich in astrocytes that create channels through which the nerve fibers pass [15]. After NRA, astrocytes proliferate and rearrange, blocking those channels and making it difficult for the regenerating nerve fibers to grow [15, 46, 56]. Axonal and dendrite regeneration is inhibited by the secretion of some substances by the astrocytes (chondroitin sulphate proteoglycans or CSPGs) [57–59] and oligodendrocytes (myelin protein [60–62] and semaphorin-3 [63]). Additionally, the glia secrete neurotoxic products like glutamate [15] and free radicals [64] that induce massive neuronal death among motor [8], sympathetic [12], parasympathetic [12] and posterior horn sensory neurons [17].

About 80% of the MNs die in the following weeks [13, 65, 66], but this death does not happen immediately after NRA [13, 67, 68]. Instead, there is a 12-day period in which different treatment strategies can reduce this MN loss [65, 69]. The chemical compounds that counteract the glutamate toxic effects can reduce the MN loss by 70%, provided that they are administered in the first 2 weeks after the NRA [16, 65, 69].

The closer the axonal injury to the neuronal body [55], the smaller the regenerating capacity of the axon and the higher the chance that the neuron will die. Four millimeters is the minimum amount of peripheral nerve that should remain to avoid MN death [70].

The surviving MNs develop axonal sprouts within 1 month after the NRA [41], but to achieve a successful regeneration, the axons must cross the gliotic TZ, grow inside the distal peripheral nerves, and reach the motor end plates [71]. The long distance to cover is a big impediment to a successful functional recovery [72, 73]. By the time the muscles get reinnervated, they are atrophic and with fibrotic changes, particularly the most distal ones [74]. The regeneration is not privative to the axon, and the dendrites can also regenerate as axon, creating what has been called a dendraxon. These also have the capacity to grow into the peripheral nerves and reinnervate muscles [75, 76].

Although the MN regenerating axon has a chance to cross the anterior SC white matter to reach its surface and then attempt to grow in a possible reimplanted NR [77, 78] for the DRG growing axon, the same is almost impossible as they have to cross a very hostile and gliotic posterior SC Dorsal Root Entry Zone (DREZ) [79–81].

In the human being, the avulsion damages more frequently the ventral NRts as they are more fragile than their posterior counterparts [15].

NRA creates four problems that have to be addressed to achieve a successful repair. First, if the axon is torn closer than 4 mm to the cell body, motor and preganglionic parasympathetic neurons undergo apoptosis [10–13, 23, 67, 68, 70, 82–84]. Second, muscles are fibrotic by the time the regenerating axonal sprouts reach the motor end plates [72, 73]. In rats, functional recovery is seen only in cervical but not in lumbosacral avulsion models as the distance to cover is much shorter for the cervical NRs [9, 40, 85–87], and in any case only proximal limb muscle recovery is seen [86–89]. Third, the regenerating fibers may reach the wrong target due to misrouting [53], and in the absence of NG or conduit, the regenerating axons will grow along the surface of the SC [27, 43, 53, 83, 87]. The misrouting is responsible for simultaneous contractures in agonist and antagonist muscles leading to ineffective limb movements [30]. Fourth, there is severe muscular atrophy due to lack of use [74]. Hence, for a successful clinical result, MN survival must be improved, axonal regeneration has to be enhanced and accelerated, misrouting should be minimized and muscle atrophy should be prevented [15, 72].

Although the MN cell body can regenerate and grow a new axon after this is torn [69, 90], many MNs apoptose [13, 65, 69], and only 80% of the surviving MNs do finally project a regenerating axon in the reimplanted ventral root or NG [26, 27, 31, 86]. Reimplantation of avulsed NRs either directly or by means of a peripheral NG helps to reduce the number of MNs undergoing apoptosis, probably because of local NF production [69, 77, 89, 91–93]. Exogenous NFs can be administered to enhance the regenerating capacity of cells [47, 94, 95].

Historically, the first attempts were directed at motor recovery with ventral rootlet reimplantantion [96], but recently sensory recovery has been proved possible by reimplanting dorsal rootlets [97]. The results of dorsal rootlet repair are dismal because the SC glial proliferation creates barriers that prevent the regenerating DRG axons from reaching the posterior SC horn [81]. The lack of sensory recovery induces chronic neuropathic pain [49, 98], and the lack of proprioception causes limb clumsiness [30]. This has been partially avoided by direct implantation of the dorsal rootlets or their NGs' extensions inside the posterior horn itself rather than on the surface of the SC [81, 99]. The repair of both motor and sensory NRts leads to better functional results with more accurate movements and less muscular synkinesis [100]. Functional MRI studies have corroborated affected limb sensory cortex function recovery in the area corresponding to the reimplanted NR [100].

The **timing of NR reimplantation** is crucial, as a longer waiting period will correlate with a greater amount of MNs undergoing apoptosis [20, 27, 91, 93, 101–103]. The percentage of dead MNs increases from 20% by 10–12 days post-avulsion [13, 65, 69] to 50% by 4 weeks [104, 105], 85% by 6 weeks [106] and 90% by 20 weeks [27, 83, 93, 107]. Early NR reimplantation seems to have neuroprotective effects [27, 83, 89, 93, 108, 109], but some MN loss will happen even if repair occurs immediately after avulsion [93, 101]. In animal models, NRA followed by immediate reimplantation in the same surgical procedure minimizes MN apoptosis and achieves muscle reinnervation with some limited functional recovery, which is better in the brachial plexus than in the lumbosacral plexus [27, 69, 83, 110]. Ideally, the surgical repair must be performed no later than 10 days post-injury [65] as a delay over 2 weeks will lead to poor clinical results [20, 26, 27]. In clinical practice, patients suffering from brachial or lumbosacral plexus avulsions often experience other concomitant injuries, sometimes quite serious, that force delaying NR repair [111]. Another common scenario is that the precise diagnosis takes weeks or even months [3]. In any case, in human beings NRA repair has to occur no later than 1 month after the injury to allow any motor function recovery [45, 74, 97, 100]. NGs are almost always needed as torn NRts retract and undergo fibrosis with time, making direct reimplantation to the SC impossible unless the repair is done just a few days after the injury [74]. This is a further difficulty as regeneration is worse with NGs than with direct NRt reimplantation [26].

3. Pharmacological aids to enhance regeneration after nerve root reimplantation

Several pharmacological aids have been introduced to improve MN survival and axonal regeneration after anterior spinal NRt reimplantation. They can be classified into NFs, drugs and cell-derived products (**Table 1**).

NF administration improves MN survival as well as synaptic and axonal regrowth [87, 112–115] improving the NR reimplantation results. NFs enhance Schwann cell migration, axonal regeneration and myelination [8, 16, 69, 93, 105, 116–120] and delay MN apoptosis—by 6 weeks 80–90% of them are still alive [8, 69, 116, 118–121]. To be maximally effective, they must be administered locally at the SC-NR interface within the first 3 days and no later than 2 weeks post-avulsion [20, 87, 93, 116]. NFs ought to be applied with Gelfoam or fibrin glue to avoid dilution in the CSF [72], but free intrathecal application by means of an injecting pump is not recommended [122]. Their short half-life limits their use, particularly because NFs have to be applied directly to a surgically exposed SC [123]. Although NFs increase MN survival and axonal regeneration, their effect on muscle recovery and final functional results is very limited [4, 7, 18, 20, 27, 37, 93, 105]. It has been observed that in areas where the concentration of NFs is high, the regenerating axons get trapped and do not grow to reach their final distal targets [18, 102]. Some have cautioned against the possible adverse effects of using NFs in human clinical practice [124]. The currently used NFs are brain-derived neurotrophic factor (BDNF) [115], glial-derived neurotrophic factor (GDNF) [8, 18, 20, 37, 102, 105, 125], ciliary neurotrophic factor (CNTF) [87] and intracellular sigma peptide (ISP) [126]. GDNF shows the strongest action and a single direct application to the SC are enough, provided that they are applied within the first 2 weeks after NRA [18, 20, 37, 102, 116, 127]. GDNF delays MN cell death for 6 weeks, therefore broadening the window for avulsed NR reimplantation [20]. Similarly, the intracellular sigma peptide (ISP) blocks astrocytic inhibitory action, thus facilitating axonal regeneration [126].

Moreover, the distance to cover by the regenerating axons from the SC avulsion site to the muscular end plates is so long that by the time the axons reach their destination, the muscles are atrophic and fibrotic [20, 128]. To avoid and delay this muscle atrophy as much as possible, several strategies have been attempted: manipulating the molecular pathways involved in muscle atrophy [129–131], nerve transfers from neighboring functioning nerves [132–136], direct electrical stimulation of the affected muscles [137–139] and neuronal transplantation inside the denervated muscle [20, 140–142]. In rats, the combination of GDNF at the SC-NR injury site and embryonic spinal foetal neuron transplant inside the target muscles provided the best possible functional result [20]. These embryonic neurons reinnervate the muscle end plates just after the injury, preventing muscle atrophy while the regenerating axons arrived

Agent	Group	Mechanism of action	Administration route	Motoneuron survival post-injury	Axonal regeneration	Observation	Applied to	Current human clinical use
Brain-derived-neurotrophic-factor (BDNF)	NF	Reverses cholinergic transmitter-related enzyme deficiency	Intrathecal	Motoneuron survival 53% by 16 weeks	Abundant regenerating fibers reaching cord-avulsed root interface	Active against many neurodegenerative disorders	Rat	None
Glial-derived-neurotrophic-factor (GDNF)	NF	⇑ Survival of dopaminergic neurons	Direct administration on spinal cord	Completely prevents motoneuron loss at 16 weeks post-avulsion	⇑ Axonal regeneration and coiling and regeneration Schwann cells	Strongest NF. ⇑ Effect combined with Riluzole Administration before 2 week post-avulsion	Rat	None
Ciliary NF (CNTF)	NF	Activates motor neuron signal transducer and transcription 3 activator(STAT3)	Direct administration on spinal cord	Motoneuron survival 23 ± 4.3% by 3 weeks post-avulsion	⇑ Axon regeneration across interface spinal cord/ nerve root	Conjugation it with transferrin prolongs its action	Rabbit	None
Intracellular sigma peptide (ISP)	NF	⇓ Inhibition of astrocyte secreted chon-droitin sulfate proteoglycans	Subcutaneous injection	Motoneuron survival 61.2% at 12 weeks post-avulsion	⇑ Amount and size of regenerated axons	Act as synapse organizing agent	Rat	None
Resveratrol	Drug	Topoisomerase II inhibitor	Added to nerve graft culture	Motoneuron survival 69% at 8 weeks post-avulsion	⇑ Axonal regeneration, Schwann cell migration and myelination	Only tried on autologous nerve graft cultures	Rat	Cancer, Chronic diseases, Aging
Riluzole	Drug	Inhibitor presynaptic glutamate release	Orally	Motoneuron survival 70% by 5 weeks post-avulsion	⇑ Myelinated axons in re-implanted nerve root. ⇓ Sensory hypersensitivity and allodynia	Administration before 2 week after injury. Maximum effect combined with GDNF	Rat	Amyotrophic lateral sclerosis, Nervous Depression, Spinal Cord Injury

http://dx.doi.org/10.5772/intechopen.82431

Agent	Group	Mechanism of action	Administration route	Motoneuron survival post-injury	Axonal regeneration	Observation	Applied to	Current human clinical use
Lithium	Drug	⇑ Endogenous BDNF secretion	Orally	Motoneuron survival 69% by 12 weeks post-avulsion	⇑ Myelinated axons inside re-implanted nerve root	Helps prevent muscle atrophy	Rat	Bipolar disorder
Minocycline	Tetracyclyne derivative	Inhibits glial proliferation. Strong anti-inflammatory effect	Orally	Motoneuron survival 48±7% at 5 weeks. Autonomic neurons ∅ effect	Improves axonal sprouting and migration	Neurotoxic at high doses. Prevents and reverses hypersensitivity	Rat, mice	Bacterial infections, Stroke
Recombinant erythropoietin	Drug	Counteracts glutamate's cytotoxic effect	Subcutaneously	Motoneuron survival $51.7 \pm 0.8\%$ at 12 days post-avulsion	Suppresses microglia proliferation. Protects axon regeneration	Induces a pro-thrombotic state. Neuroprotective effect NOT long-lasting	Rat	Anemia
FK506-tacrolimus	Drug	Immunosuppression. Target heat shock protein 90	Sublingual	Motoneuron survival not reported. Used ONLY in dorsal nerve root repair	⇑ Regenerating axons penetrating and reaching the posterior horn	Immunosuppression. Long-term administration needed	Rat	Organ transplant immunosuppression
Geldamycin	Ansamycin antibiotic	On heat shock protein 90. NOT immunosuppression	Parenteral injection	⇑ Survival dorsal ganglion neuron. Motoneuron not studied	Accelerates axonal regeneration	No immunosuppression. Toxic at high doses	Rat	Cancer
Acamprosate	Drug	⇓ Synaptic glutamate	Orally	Associated with ribavirin ⇑	Associated with ribavirin accelerates	Side effects if ethanol consumption	Rat	Alcoholism

Agent	Group	Mechanism of action	Administration route	Motoneuron survival post-injury	Axonal regeneration	Observation	Applied to	Current human clinical use
				motoneuron survival by 64.62% at 1 week	axonal regeneration >4 weeks			
Ribavirin	Drug	Synthetic guanosine antiviral properties	Orally	Associated with acamprosate ⇑ motoneuron survival by 64.62% at 1 week	Associated with Acamprosate accelerates axonal regeneration >4 weeks	Can induce anemia	Rat	Hepatitis virus C
N-acetyl cysteine	Drug	Stabilizes oxidative metabolism	Orally	Neuron survival 26% motor, 95% sensory	Facilitates axonal regeneration	Vitamin C counteracts side effects	Rat	Mucolytic
Glatiramer	Drug	Immunomodulator	Subcutaneously	⇑ Motoneuron survival but NOT quantified	Reduction in astrocyte proliferation	⇑ Risk of infection and malignancy	Rat	Multiple sclerosis

Table 1. NFs (neurotrophic factors) and drugs used in nerve root reimplantation with their effects.

[20]. However, when the regenerating axons reached the muscular end plates, they had to compete with the already existing axons coming from the locally injected embryonic foetal neurons [20, 140, 143, 144].

Some **drugs** have been administered **to minimize MN apoptosis and improve NR regeneration**: resveratrol (3,4′,5-trihydroxystilbene) [145], riluzole (2-amino-6-trifluoromethoxybenzothiazole) [8, 69, 121], lithium [146, 147], minocycline [119], recombinant erythropoietin [118], FK506-tacrolimus [148–151], geldanamycin [152, 153], acamprosate [67, 154], ribavirin [154], N-acetyl cysteine [155] and glatiramer [156]. Some researchers have administered combinations such as acamprosate and ribavirin [154] or riluzole and GDNF [8]. The main advantage of acamprosate, ribavirin, and riluzole is that they can be administered orally [67, 154, 157].

Resveratrol has been added to the autologous NG culture for a week in the rat experimental C_6 NRA and reimplantation model [145], finding that it improves axonal regeneration, Schwann cell migration and myelination and MN survival—69% surviving 8 weeks after NR repair.

In experimental brachial plexus avulsion (BPA) rat models, **riluzole** has been proved to improve MN survival, prolonging the time period at which reimplantation can be successful [65, 69, 101, 121]. If administered within 2 weeks post-avulsion, riluzole helps to keep 70% of the MNs [65, 69, 121] alive and minimizes the sensory hypersensitivity and allodynia [119]. Its maximum effect is achieved when combined with GDNF [8], and it can be administered orally [157].

In rat, experimental avulsion models and at doses used in the treatment of mood disorders, **lithium** improves neuronal survival, axonal regeneration and myelination, allowing an earlier and better functional recovery [146, 147]. One of its mechanisms of action is by increasing endogenous BDNF secretion [158]. Its effect on growing axon myelination starts 4 weeks post-NR reimplantation, reaching its pinnacle at 6 weeks and slowing down by 12 weeks [146].

Minocycline is a tetracycline derivative that inhibits glial proliferation [159]—a barrier against axonal and dendrite growth [160]—and decreases neuronal [161] and oligodendrocyte cell loss [120, 162, 163]. Minocycline can cross the blood–brain barrier and has anti-inflammatory properties [120]. In rats, it has been administered intraperitoneally and intrathecally, with better results through the latter route [106]. At low doses, minocycline has neuroprotective properties, but at high concentrations it is neurotoxic [164], among other reasons, because glial proliferation and Wallerian degeneration are a *sine qua non* for nerve regeneration [106].

Recombinant erythropoietin injected subcutaneously once a day for 3 days has shown neuroprotective properties in a rat NRA experimental model [118]. These neuroprotective properties are short lasting but can help to delay motor neuron apoptosis after NRA, increasing the period in which a NR reimplantation can be undertaken [118]. Recombinant erythropoietin seems to counteract the cytotoxic effect of glutamate, block free radicals, increase the release of neurotransmitters and decrease microglial activation [165]. The positive effects of recombinant erythropoietin are maximal when its administration is started within 96 hours (4 days) after NRA and reimplantation [118]. The side effects related with the administration of this drug—increase in erythrocyte production and a prothrombotic state—are not problematic because this drug is only administered for 3 days [118]. Perhaps administering this drug for a longer period of time could provide additional neuroprotective effects, but 3 days are enough to prolong the period in which a successful NR reimplantation can be performed [118].

FK506-tacrolimus improved the amount of regenerating posterior NR axons penetrating the SC and reaching the posterior horn [151].

Acamprosate is a taurine analogue used to prevent relapse in alcoholic patients that acts as neuroprotective and accelerates axonal regeneration [154, 166].

Ribavirin is a nucleoside antimetabolite antiviral agent that blocks nucleic acid synthesis that is administered together with acamprosate to encourage axonal regeneration [154].

N-Acetyl cysteine administered intraperitoneally and intrathecally in rats enhances the rate of MN survival and facilitates regeneration in case of NR reimplantation [155].

Glatiramer is a polymer of L-alanine, L-glutamic acid, L-lysine and L-tyrosine that structurally resembles the myelin basic protein and that when administered daily reduces the gliosis and the avulsed MN synaptic stripping [156].

To summarize, in NRA reimplantation GDGF applied directly to the anterior SC—to the point where the motor rootlets go out—associated with oral riluzole provides the highest rate of MN survival and axonal regeneration [8]. For the dorsal root, CNTF [87] applied directly to the section of the posterior SC where the sensory rootlets get in combined with oral N-acetyl cysteine [155] allows maximal sensory neuron survival. Other agents could be added, such as oral minocycline [106, 120], tacrolimus [151] or recombinant erythropoietin [118, 165]to reduce the reactive glial proliferation that impairs the axonal regeneration. ISP should be administered subcutaneously to minimize astrocyte inhibition of axonal regeneration [126, 167]. The data are summarized in **Table 1**.

Another strategy has been to apply **pluripotent cells** at the SC avulsion site to improve MN survival and axonal regeneration. These have been particularly useful in minimizing neuronal apoptosis. Among them are induced pluripotent stem cells (iPSC) [143], mesenchymal stem cells (MSCs) [168–170], olfactory ensheathing glial cells (OECs) [85, 171], bone marrow stem cells (BMC) [172], human fibroblast growth factor 2 (FGG2) [95], neuroectodermal stem cells (ESC) [143], murine neural crest stem cells (MNCSC) [173], embryonic stem cell-derived neuron precursors (ESCDNP) [173] and neural progenitor cells (NPC) [140, 141, 168, 174]. The human embryonic stem cells overexpressing human fibroblast growth factor 2 (FGG2) applied at the injury site improved MN survival and reduced the glial reactivity, thus improving the regenerating capacities [95]. However, it has unknown effectivity, only shown in animal experimental studies, and its application in the human being creates ethical issues.

Some researchers have found in vivo that a week time gap between NG harvest and its subsequent use in nerve repair improves the regenerating capacities [175] by increasing the number of Schwann cells and macrophages inside the NG [145, 176, 177] as well as by inducing the local GDNF release [145, 178, 179]. This is another possibility but difficult to use in clinical practice.

A word of caution is to be said about the **materials used to glue the peripheral NGs to the SC**. Only Tisseel® causes no long-term histological reaction [180, 181], while other preparations available in the market (BioGlue®, Adherus®) induce local fibrous reaction with SC adherences and at times neurological sequelae [181]. BioGlue® when applied close or in contact with nervous tissues can create serious damages [182]. In rats, some researchers have used snake (*Crotalus durissus terrificus*) venom-derived fibrin glue and reported excellent results [183, 184]. In clinical practice, fibrin glue from human origin is usually used [15, 30, 33, 45, 185].

On the other hand, conduits can be used to substitute autologous NGs. They have been extensively tried in peripheral nerve repairs [186, 187], but in NR reimplantation the data available are more limited [188, 189]. In peripheral nerve repair, these conduits have proved useful up to distances of 70 mm in length [37, 38, 190]. Certainly, the central-peripheral nervous tissue interface is a place in which autologous NFs provided by the autologous NGs play a pivotal role in regeneration of the reimplanted NR [69, 77, 89, 91–93]. Some researchers have tried nerve conduits enriched with BDNF that have had a good result in a rabbit experimental model [191]. In human clinical practice, there are currently no published reports [45, 74].

However, the applicability of all these studies is limited since they were generated with experimental animal models and with reimplantation immediately following the avulsion. On top of that, the regenerating capacities of the human nervous system are much less than that observed in research animals (the rat especially [73]), and the reimplantation of an avulsed NR has to be delayed weeks or even months until the patient is stabilized from other traumatic lesions and when an adequate diagnosis and treatment strategy are well defined [111].

4. Surgical technique of human NR reimplantation

Surgical techniques can be useful, particularly in complete BPA and with a delay between the injury and the surgical repair of no longer than 4 weeks [45]. Some significant problems are that MN apoptosis is greater as the time goes by [20, 27, 91, 93, 101–103] and that by 4 weeks, there is a dense scar around the BP as well as the avulsed NRs and in their intervertebral foramina that hinders any surgical manoeuvres [45, 74].

The surgical approaches described can be summarized into posterior subscapular [192], lateral [193], anterolateral [194, 195] and single-stage combined anterior (first) and posterior (second) [33].

4.1. Posterior subscapular approach

With the patient in the prone position, a longitudinal incision is made halfway between the spine and the scapula [39, 192, 196]. The trapezius muscle is sectioned transversally in the direction of its fibers. The rhomboid major and minor muscles are also divided following the direction of their fibers. The T_1 transverse process is identified and removed with the aid of a drill. A section of the first rib is also removed. A laminectomy and facetectomy are needed to access the spinal canal. The dura is opened and the dentate ligaments sectioned to rotate the SC to reach the implantation site of the ventral roots. As no access to the anterior structures is possible, another anterior approach to the BP is needed to identify and mobilize it and to pass the NGs from one surgical field to the other [7]. Depending on the degree of bone removal, a posterior cervical fusion might be required. This approach only allows access to the avulsed NRs that lie inside the spinal canal or outside it but very close to the foramina [39]. Only one case was reported in 1995 [39], which did not spark much interest within the BP surgical community. Currently this technique is not used for NR reimplantation.

4.2. Lateral approach

This has been well described in the publications of Carlstedt and co-authors [7, 44, 45, 193]. The patient is placed on the lateral decubitus position with the affected arm at the highest position and slightly rotated outwards with the hand in supination. The head is supported in a Mayfield head clamp (Integra LifeSciences, Austin, Texas, USA) and, slightly laterally, bent towards the healthy side. The idea is not only to allow surgical access to the whole BP but also to the possible donor sensory nerves (median antebrachial cutaneous and radial sensory nerves). The ipsilateral lower limb saphenous nerve can also be accessed with ease. The surgical table is placed in a 15% head-up position to reduce venous bleeding. A skin incision is performed from the mastoid to the clavicle following the posterior border of the sternocleidomastoid muscle [7, 44, 45],or by incising from the sternocleidomastoid muscle-clavicular incision and running parallel to the clavicle about 2 cm above it in the direction of the C_7 spinous process [193]. After dissecting the platysma and sternocleidomastoid muscles, the spinal accessory and cervical plexus nerves are identified and referenced with loops. Care has to be taken not to damage the spinal accessory nerve at the junction between the upper and middle-third sternocleidomastoid muscle posterior border. After careful subcutaneous fat dissection, the transverse processes of the cervical vertebrae can be felt deep to the sternocleidomastoid muscle with the tip of the finger. The scalene muscles anterior, middle and posterior as well as the levator scapula muscle are identified. Next, the transverse cervical artery and vein are isolated and referenced. It is best not to sacrifice them as they can be used in the future to vascularise a possible gracilis muscle graft [197]. The BP is fully exposed and the avulsed NRs identified. The avulsed NRs are trimmed until normal-appearing nervous tissue is seen. Many surgeons remove the dorsal root including its ganglion [15, 45]. Unless the NR reimplantation is attempted in the first 2 weeks post-avulsion injury, the BP retracts distally and undergoes fibrotic changes adhering to the nearby structures [1, 26, 33, 198, 199], so the BP has to be completely freed to be able to move it upwards. This maneuver can be troublesome at times due to dense fibrotic tissue, particularly when surgical reimplantation has been delayed over 4 weeks [15, 45]. When this is not possible or the BP cannot regain its former position in contralateral C_7 NR transfer, some have shortened the humerus shaft by 4 cm [198]. The alternative is to use long autologous NGs that cover the gap between the SC and the NR remnants [15, 26, 45, 109].

The C_5-T_1 NR foramina and zygapophyseal joints are approached between the elevator scapula and the middle and posterior scalene muscles. Then the *longissimus* muscle is split longitudinally to expose the spine. The *multifidus* muscles are detached from the zygapophyseal joints

http://dx.doi.org/10.5772/intechopen.82431

and laminae. The transverse processes and the anterior and posterior tubercles are exposed by removing all the muscles attaching to them. These bone structures plus a section of the lateral mass are removed and a C5-C7 hemilaminectomy performed. The removed bone pieces are saved for later use.

Care must be taken with the vertebral artery, as it does not need to be mobilized. As most of the lateral mass, the disc and the contralateral facet joints are spared; the procedure usually does not induce spine instability. The avulsed NRs can be identified by pseudomeningoceles. The C_5–C_7 foramina are exposed with ease, while the C_8 and T_1 are much more difficult, and some surgeons refuse to do it to concentrate in repairing only the C_5–C_7 NRs, even if the lower ones are also damaged [45]. This is important because no improvement can be expected in roots that have never been reimplanted and explains one of the reasons why the distal muscles of the hand are seldom reinnervated [15, 45]. Some researchers have proven in rat experimental studies that a single reimplanted NR can attract regenerating axonal sprouts from nearby levels [200].

The dura mater is exposed and opened longitudinally and the dentate ligaments sectioned. Intraoperative neurophysiological monitoring is recommended particularly on rotating the SC and when performing the longitudinal myelotomy and inserting the NGs inside it [45].

4.2.1. Ventral root repair

The SC is rotated, pulling from the dentate ligaments to expose its anterior aspect. Serial 2–3 mm-long stab incisions are done at the same place where the anterior NRs formerly stood. Peripheral nerve sensory NGs (medial antebrachial cutaneous nerve, superficial radial nerve, saphenous nerve) are introduced 1 mm inside the SC tissue [201] and secured with Tisseel fibrin glue (Immuno AG, Vienna, Austria). The distal stumps of these NGs are sutured with the corresponding avulsed NR remnant. The dura mater is repaired with a dural substitute and the suture reinforced with fibrin glue to prevent CSF leaks.

Some anatomical studies have found that the best spot where to insert the NGs in the SC is where the anterior NRs formerly stood and not in the lateral SC side [201]. This latter place is technically easier and achieves some regeneration by lateral MN axon sprouting, but the results are inadequate [201]. As the NG implantation inside the SC will cause a further damage to it [26], suturing the NGs to the SC pial surface in an experimental avulsion model has been tried, finding that it allows adequate MN survival and axonal regeneration [27]. This ventral root pial reimplantation is not only less risky but technically easier [26, 33].

4.2.2. Dorsal rootlet repair

This was first reported in 1997 in an experimental rat NRA model [202]. Peripheral NGs were used to cover the gap between the remaining dorsal NR and the SC. A DREZ longitudinal myelotomy was performed to insert the NGs 2 mm inside the posterior horn. Some regeneration was seen with peroxidase staining [202]. The addition of olfactory ensheathing cells at the DREZ in 2003 did not improve the results [171]. In 2004, Tang et al. [188] also in rats used bioresorbable nerve conduits to repair a 6 mm dorsal NR gap, showing signs of recovery. This repair was enhanced by injecting a viral vector inside the DRG [203]. In 2017, Konig et al. [173] reported the application of murine neural crest stem cells and embryonic stem cell-derived neuron precursors at the DREZ in an experimental rat cervical dorsal NRA showing differentiation into neurons and their migration, transforming into interneurons and facilitating the creation of synapsis with the regenerating axons coming from the reimplanted dorsal NR.

In humans, dorsal rootlet repair has been recently attempted by Carlstedt et al. [97]. As they noticed the extreme difficulty for the growing axons coming from the DRG to cross the glial scar at the surface of the posterior horn, they sectioned the avulsed NR distal to the DRG and sutured the peripheral sensory stump to the posterior horn by means of NGs introduced in the SC through a longitudinal myelotomy. The rationale was to get some sensory recovery from the growing axons of the posterior horn neurons that are expected to grow distally inside the implanted NG [99]. As the neuronal bodies of the DRG are removed, the regeneration has to depend on the neuronal plasticity of neurons coming from the posterior horn that have to stretch their axons to reach the skin though the NGs and peripheral nerves. The results are poor [99, 100], but it is the first strategy that has provided some success in humans. This is not ideal as sensation could be recovered if the dorsal rootlets were replaced by NGs and the tip of those grafts inserted inside the posterior SC horn through a longitudinal myelotomy while maintaining the neuronal bodies that lie at the DRG. This technique proved effective in rats [202], but no attempts in humans have been found in the literature. To improve the results, CNTF [87] should apply locally to the posterior SC at the DREZ associated with N-acetyl cysteine [155] *orally* to allow maximal sensory neuron survival. Oral minocycline [106, 120], oral tacrolimus [151] or subcutaneous recombinant erythropoietin [118, 165] could be also administered to reduce the reactive glial proliferation that acts as a barrier against dorsal root axonal regeneration.

4.2.3. Wound closure

The dura mater is closed with a dural substitute and reinforced with fibrin glue to prevent CSF leaks. The morcellized bone obtained from the transverse processes and lateral masses supplemented together with demineralized bone matrix is laid on the cervical spinal column defect to enhance bone fusion. A lumbar drain is inserted and kept for 5 days to prevent CSF leaks.

Postoperatively, patients are kept with a sling for 6 weeks before starting any passive movements, to prevent NG dislodgement [45]. Cervical X-rays are taken every 3 months for a year to detect any possible instability that might require a cervical fusion.

The most important disadvantage of this approach is that it entails extensive muscular damage, particularly at the scalene muscles [33]. The most significant advantage is that the NGs needed for the repair are the shortest of all the NRA reimplantation approaches [45, 193].

4.3. Anterolateral approach

It is first described by George et al. for the treatment of cervical spinal spondylosis and tumors [204, 205]. This approach is much more direct but demands a partial multilevel oblique partial

http://dx.doi.org/10.5772/intechopen.82431

corpectomy of the affected levels that can be C_4 to T_1 when the whole BP is involved. This involves an extensive anterior cervical fusion, not optimal for younger individuals due to its possible long-term consequences [206]. The anterolateral approach provides good access to the BP and ventral NR, but the dorsal NR cannot be reimplanted [195]. This approach has been reported in research animals—cats [207, 208]—in ten cadavers and four clinical cases [194], but no long-term clinical results have been reported.

4.4. Single-stage combined anterior (first) and posterior (second) approach

The antecedent of this approach is the **two-stage combined approach posterior (first) and anterior (some days later)** [185]. In the first stage, the cervical spinal canal was approached with the patient prone. A C_4–T_1 laminectomy with medial-third facetectomy was performed and the SC inspected after longitudinal dural opening. The dentate ligaments were sectioned and SC rotated and inspected looking for avulsed NR. In case the avulsed NRts were inside the dura mater, they were reimplanted where they formerly stood. Both ventral and dorsal NRs were reimplanted. When the NRs were outside the spinal canal, NGs were inserted and sutured to the SC tissue through small myelotomies and their distal end tunneled through the paraspinal muscles and placed in the supraclavicular area with two metallic hemoclips to facilitate their identification in the future. The dura mater was sutured and sealed with fibrin glue. A posterior mass cervical fusion was performed to prevent postoperative kyphotic deformities. Some days later the patient was taken back to the operating room and in the supine position the BP identified and isolated in the supraclavicular region. The NG distal ends were localized through the hemoclips with X-ray guidance and sutured to the corresponding BP cords. Apart from the original report [116], no further publications on this seem to exist.

The **single-stage combined anterior (first) and posterior (second) approach** was reported by Amr el al. in 2009 [33]. The patient is placed in the lateral decubitus position and the skin sterilized front and back of neck and chest as well as the whole affected upper limb and both lower limbs. Then the patient is rotated backwards and placed supine. In this position a traditional BP exploration is done through a transverse supraclavicular incision. If needed, a second incision perpendicular to it can be done following the delto-pectoral groove. This allows exploration of the infra-clavicular BP, particularly when it has migrated distally. Once the whole BP is dissected free and the damages evaluated, several peripheral sensory NGs are obtained from the affected upper limb and both lower limbs. These grafts are sutured to the cords of the avulsed NR.

Next, the patient is placed again in the lateral position. Through a posterior midline incision from occiput to T_2, the whole cervical spine is exposed. The spinal muscles are detached from the spinous process and separated laterally. A laminectomy and partial medial facetectomy C_4–T_1 are performed on the affected side. The dura is opened through a longitudinal incision and the dentate ligaments sectioned. The NG that had been previously sutured to the BP cords in an end-to-side versus end-to-end technique [33, 209] is passed subcutaneously from the anterior surgical field to the laminectomy area. These NG needs to be long enough to cover the distance between the SC and the BP. Then the proximal ends of the NGs are sutured subpially in a longitudinal fashion, parallel to the side where the ventral roots stood. No SC incisions are performed. The proximal ends of the NGs are sutured intradurally to C_4 above and to T_1 below. In the only publication that we have found, the dorsal NRs are not repaired [33]. The dura is closed with interrupted stitches reinforced with fibrin glue. No cervical fusion is applied.

The advantage of this double approach is that it is more conservative to the muscles. The disadvantage is that long NGs are needed, making the distance between the motoneuron and the muscular end plates still larger. To the best of our knowledge, there is only a single publication attesting the validity of this technique [33]. It is of particular interest that ventral NR regeneration can be achieved by laying the NGs subpially at the SC without having to insert them inside the SC tissue through myelotomies [33].

5. Clinical results in human beings

Some clinical studies have reported definitive although limited motor and sensory improvements particularly in the proximal limb areas after NR reimplantation in complete BPAs [15, 30, 32, 33, 45, 185]. The best motor recovery was seen at the deltoid, pectoralis, infraspinatus, biceps and triceps muscles [15, 30, 45, 185, 209]. One patient showed signs of partial recovery of the flexor digitorum superficialis and another of the first dorsal interosseous muscle [45]. A functional recovery of the hand has only been reported in a 9-year-old child with a complete BPA [29]. Hand intrinsic muscle motor grade 2 recovery was reported by Amr et al. [33]. The best sensory improvement was patent at dermatomes C_5, C_6 and T_1, particularly at C_5 [33, 45]. One of the reasons by which only proximal muscles show signs of reinnervation in the work of Kachramanoglou et al. is because only the C_5–C_7 NRs are reimplanted as C_8 and T_1 are more technically demanding and they were reluctant to risk neurological complications on handling the SC at these levels [45]. This could also be the reason by which Amr et al. [33] report hand intrinsic muscle grade 2 motor recovery, as they did repair the C_8 and T_1 roots. Another extremely important reason is that when the regenerating axons reach the distal limb muscles, they are already atrophied and fibrotic [72, 73]. The C_5 and T_1 sensory recovery can in part be due to overlapping sensory covering from nearby dermatomes (C_4 for C_5 and T_2 for T_1) [32, 45].

6. Conclusions

NRA keeps being in an area in which improvement is desperately needed, particularly in complete BPAs in which not many alternatives are possible. As clinical results in humans keep being dismal, further research is needed. The administration of drugs, preferably orally, has to be pursued to find a combination of them that helps to achieve a successful limb recovery. NR reimplantation has to be undertaken as soon as the patients' clinical condition allows it. Ventral NRt implantation provides better results than its posterior counterparts.

http://dx.doi.org/10.5772/intechopen.82431

Abbreviations

BDNF	brain-derived neurotrophic factor
BMC	bone marrow stem cells
BP	brachial plexus
BPA	brachial plexus avulsion
CNF	ciliary neurotrophic factor
GDNF	glial-derived neurotrophic factor
iPSC	induced pluripotent stem cells
ISP	intracellular sigma peptide
MN	motor neuron
MSCs	mesenchymal stem cells
NF	neurotrophic factor
NGs	nerve grafts
NPC	neural progenitor cells
NR	nerve root
NRA	nerve root avulsion
NRts	nerve rootlets
NSC	neuroectodermal stem cells
OECs	olfactory ensheathing glial cells
SC	spinal cord

Author details

Vicente Vanaclocha-Vanaclocha[1]*, Nieves Saiz-Sapena[2], José María Ortiz-Criado[3] and Leyre Vanaclocha[4]

*Address all correspondence to: vvanaclo@hotmail.com

1 Hospital General Universitario Valencia, Spain

2 Hospital 9 de Octubre, Valencia, Spain

3 Universidad Católica San Vicente Mártir, Valencia, Spain

4 Medical School, University College London, London, United Kingdom

References

[1] Abou-Al-Shaar H, Karsy M, Ravindra V, Joyce E, Mahan MA. Acute repair of traumatic pan-brachial plexus injury: Technical considerations and approaches. Neurosurgical Focus. 2018;**44**(VideoSuppl1):V4. DOI: 10.3171/2018.1.FocusVid.17569

[2] Barman A, Chatterjee A, Prakash H, Viswanathan A, Tharion G, Thomas R. Traumatic brachial plexus injury: Electrodiagnostic findings from 111 patients in a tertiary care hospital in India. Injury. 2012;**43**(11):1943-1948. DOI: 10.1016/j.injury.2012.07.182

[3] Bertelli JA, Ghizoni MF, Soldado F. Patterns of brachial plexus stretch palsy in a prospective series of 565 surgically treated patients. Journal of Hand Surgery. 2017;**42**(6):443-446.e2. DOI: 10.1016/j.jhsa.2017.03.021

[4] Hoffmann CF, Thomeer RT, Marani E. Reimplantation of ventral rootlets into the cervical spinal cord after their avulsion: An anterior surgical approach. Clinical Neurology and Neurosurgery. 1993;**95**(Suppl):S112-S118

[5] Okby R, Sheiner E. Risk factors for neonatal brachial plexus paralysis. Archives of Gynecology and Obstetrics. 2012;**286**(2):333-336. DOI: 10.1007/s00404-012-2272-z

[6] Chambers JA, Hiles CL, Keene BP. Brachial plexus injury management in military casualties: Who, what, when, why, and how. Military Medicine. 2014;**179**(6):640-644. DOI: 10.7205/MILMED-D-13-00457

[7] Carlstedt T, Anand P, Hallin R, Misra PV, Norén G, Seferlis T. Spinal nerve root repair and reimplantation of avulsed ventral roots into the spinal cord after brachial plexus injury. Journal of Neurosurgery. 2000;**93**(2 Suppl):237-247

[8] Bergerot A, Shortland PJ, Anand P, Hunt SP, Carlstedt T. Co-treatment with riluzole and GDNF is necessary for functional recovery after ventral root avulsion injury. Experimental Neurology. 2004;**187**(2):359-366. DOI: 10.1016/j.expneurol.2004.02.003

[9] Ruven C, Chan T-K, Wu W. Spinal root avulsion: An excellent model for studying motoneuron degeneration and regeneration after severe axonal injury. Neural Regeneration Research. 2014;**9**(2):117-118. DOI: 10.4103/1673-5374.125338

[10] Martin LJ, Kaiser A, Price AC. Motor neuron degeneration after sciatic nerve avulsion in adult rat evolves with oxidative stress and is apoptosis. Journal of Neurobiology. 1999; **40**(2):185-201

[11] Martin LJ, Liu Z. Injury-induced spinal motor neuron apoptosis is preceded by DNA single-strand breaks and is p53- and Bax-dependent. Journal of Neurobiology. 2002;**50**(3): 181-197

[12] Hoang TX, Nieto JH, Tillakaratne NJK, Havton LA. Autonomic and motor neuron death is progressive and parallel in a lumbosacral ventral root avulsion model of cauda equina injury. The Journal of Comparative Neurology. 2003;**467**(4):477-486. DOI: 10.1002/cne.10928

[13] Koliatsos VE, Price WL, Pardo CA, Price DL. Ventral root avulsion: An experimental model of death of adult motor neurons. The Journal of Comparative Neurology. 1994; **342**(1):35-44. DOI: 10.1002/cne.903420105

[14] Havton LA, Carlstedt T. Repair and rehabilitation of plexus and root avulsions in animal models and patients. Current Opinion in Neurology. 2009;**22**(6):570-574. DOI: 10.1097/WCO.0b013e328331b63f

[15] Carlstedt T. Root repair review: Basic science background and clinical outcome. Restorative Neurology and Neuroscience. 2008;**26**(2-3):225-241

[16] Nógrádi A, Vrbová G. Improved motor function of denervated rat hindlimb muscles induced by embryonic spinal cord grafts. The European Journal of Neuroscience. 1996; **8**(10):2198-2203

[17] Chew DJ, Leinster VHL, Sakthithasan M, Robson LG, Carlstedt T, Shortland PJ. Cell death after dorsal root injury. Neuroscience Letters. 2008;**433**(3):231-234. DOI: 10.1016/j.neulet.2008.01.012

[18] Blits B, Carlstedt TP, Ruitenberg MJ, et al. Rescue and sprouting of motoneurons following ventral root avulsion and reimplantation combined with intraspinal adeno-associated viral vector-mediated expression of glial cell line-derived neurotrophic factor or brain-derived neurotrophic factor. Experimental Neurology. 2004;**189**(2):303-316. DOI: 10.1016/j.expneurol.2004.05.014

[19] Bertelli JA, Ghizoni MF. Reconstruction of C5 and C6 brachial plexus avulsion injury by multiple nerve transfers: Spinal accessory to suprascapular, ulnar fascicles to biceps branch, and triceps long or lateral head branch to axillary nerve. Journal of Hand Surgery. 2004;**29**(1):131-139

[20] Ruven C, Badea S-R, Wong W-M, Wu W. Combination treatment with exogenous GDNF and fetal spinal cord cells results in better Motoneuron survival and functional recovery after avulsion injury with delayed root reimplantation. Journal of Neuropathology and Experimental Neurology. 2018;**77**(4):325-343. DOI: 10.1093/jnen/nly009

[21] Jeanmonod D, Sindou M, Mauguière F. Intraoperative electrophysiological recordings during microsurgical DREZ-tomies in man. Stereotactic and Functional Neurosurgery. 1990;**54-55**:80-85. DOI: 10.1159/000100195

[22] Guenot M, Hupe JM, Mertens P, Ainsworth A, Bullier J, Sindou M. A new type of microelectrode for obtaining unitary recordings in the human spinal cord. Journal of Neurosurgery. 1999;**91**(1 Suppl):25-32

[23] Carlstedt T, Havton L. The longitudinal spinal cord injury: lessons from intraspinal plexus, cauda equina and medullary conus lesions. Handbook of Clinical Neurology. 2012;**109**:337-354. DOI: 10.1016/B978-0-444-52137-8.00021-8

[24] Htut M, Misra P, Anand P, Birch R, Carlstedt T. Pain phenomena and sensory recovery following brachial plexus avulsion injury and surgical repairs. Journal of Hand Surgery (Edinburgh, Scotland). 2006;**31**(6):596-605. DOI: 10.1016/j.jhsb.2006.04.027

[25] Vredeveld JW, Blaauw G, Slooff BA, Richards R, Rozeman SC. The findings in paediatric obstetric brachial palsy differ from those in older patients: A suggested explanation. Developmental Medicine and Child Neurology. 2000;**42**(3):158-161

[26] Su H, Yuan Q, Qin D, et al. Ventral root re-implantation is better than peripheral nerve transplantation for motoneuron survival and regeneration after spinal root avulsion injury. BMC Surgery. 2013;**13**:21. DOI: 10.1186/1471-2482-13-21

[27] Gu H-Y, Chai H, Zhang J-Y, et al. Survival, regeneration and functional recovery of motoneurons after delayed reimplantation of avulsed spinal root in adult rat. Experimental Neurology. 2005;**192**(1):89-99. DOI: 10.1016/j.expneurol.2004.10.019

[28] Chuang T-Y, Huang M-C, Chen K-C, et al. Forelimb muscle activity following nerve graft repair of ventral roots in the rat cervical spinal cord. Life Sciences. 2002;**71**(5):487-496

[29] Carlstedt T, Anand P, Htut M, Misra P, Svensson M. Restoration of hand function and so called "breathing arm" after intraspinal repair of C5-T1 brachial plexus avulsion injury. Case report. Neurosurgical Focus. 2004;**16**(5):E7

[30] Htut M, Misra VP, Anand P, Birch R, Carlstedt T. Motor recovery and the breathing arm after brachial plexus surgical repairs, including re-implantation of avulsed spinal roots into the spinal cord. The Journal of Hand Surgery, European Volume. 2007;**32**(2):170-178. DOI: 10.1016/J.JHSB.2006.11.011

[31] Wu W, Chai H, Zhang J, Gu H, Xie Y, Zhou L. Delayed implantation of a peripheral nerve graft reduces motoneuron survival but does not affect regeneration following spinal root avulsion in adult rats. Journal of Neurotrauma. 2004;**21**(8):1050-1058. DOI: 10.1089/0897715041651006

[32] Bertelli JA, Ghizoni MF. Brachial plexus avulsion injury repairs with nerve transfers and nerve grafts directly implanted into the spinal cord yield partial recovery of shoulder and elbow movements. Neurosurgery. 2003;**52**(6):1385-1389-1390

[33] Amr SM, Essam AM, Abdel-Meguid AMS, Kholeif AM, Moharram AN, El-Sadek RER. Direct cord implantation in brachial plexus avulsions: Revised technique using a single stage combined anterior (first) posterior (second) approach and end-to-side side-to-side grafting neurorrhaphy. Journal of Brachial Plexus and Peripheral Nerve Injury. 2009;**4**:8. DOI: 10.1186/1749-7221-4-8

[34] Nichols CM, Brenner MJ, Fox IK, et al. Effects of motor versus sensory nerve grafts on peripheral nerve regeneration. Experimental Neurology. 2004;**190**(2):347-355. DOI: 10.1016/j.expneurol.2004.08.003

[35] Chu T-H, Du Y, Wu W. Motor nerve graft is better than sensory nerve graft for survival and regeneration of motoneurons after spinal root avulsion in adult rats. Experimental Neurology. 2008;**212**(2):562-565. DOI: 10.1016/j.expneurol.2008.05.001

[36] Lin Y-L, Chang K-T, Lin C-T, et al. Repairing the ventral root is sufficient for simultaneous motor and sensory recovery in multiple complete cervical root transection injuries. Life Sciences. 2014;**109**(1):44-49. DOI: 10.1016/j.lfs.2014.06.001

[37] Chu T-H, Wang L, Guo A, Chan VW-K, Wong CW-M, Wu W. GDNF-treated acellular nerve graft promotes motoneuron axon regeneration after implantation into cervical root avulsed spinal cord. Neuropathology and Applied Neurobiology. 2012;**38**(7):681-695. DOI: 10.1111/j.1365-2990.2012.01253.x

[38] Kassar-Duchossoy L, Duchossoy Y, Rhrich-Haddout F, Horvat JC. Reinnervation of a denervated skeletal muscle by spinal axons regenerating through a collagen channel directly implanted into the rat spinal cord. Brain Research. 2001;**908**(1):25-34

[39] Carlstedt T, Grane P, Hallin RG, Norén G. Return of function after spinal cord implantation of avulsed spinal nerve roots. Lancet Lond Engl. 1995;**346**(8986):1323-1325

[40] Carlstedt T, Lindå H, Cullheim S, Risling M. Reinnervation of hind limb muscles after ventral root avulsion and implantation in the lumbar spinal cord of the adult rat. Acta Physiologica Scandinavica. 1986;**128**(4):645-646. DOI: 10.1111/j.1748-1716.1986.tb08024.x

[41] Cullheim S, Carlstedt T, Lindå H, Risling M, Ulfhake B. Motoneurons reinnervate skeletal muscle after ventral root implantation into the spinal cord of the cat. Neuroscience. 1989;**29**(3):725-733

[42] Carlstedt TP, Hallin RG, Hedström KG, Nilsson-Remahl IA. Functional recovery in primates with brachial plexus injury after spinal cord implantation of avulsed ventral roots. Journal of Neurology, Neurosurgery, and Psychiatry. 1993;**56**(6):649-654

[43] Hallin RG, Carlstedt T, Nilsson-Remahl I, Risling M. Spinal cord implantation of avulsed ventral roots in primates; correlation between restored motor function and morphology. Experimental Brain Research. 1999;**124**(3):304-310

[44] Carlstedt T, Norén G. Repair of ruptured spinal nerve roots in a brachial plexus lesion. Case report. Journal of Neurosurgery. 1995;**82**(4):661-663. DOI: 10.3171/jns.1995.82.4.0661

[45] Kachramanoglou C, Carlstedt T, Koltzenburg M, Choi D. Long-term outcome of brachial plexus reimplantation after complete brachial plexus avulsion injury. World Neurosurgery. 2017;**103**:28-36. DOI: 10.1016/j.wneu.2017.03.052

[46] Fraher JP. The transitional zone and CNS regeneration. Journal of Anatomy. 2000;**196** (Pt 1):137-158

[47] Madduri S, Gander B. Schwann cell delivery of neurotrophic factors for peripheral nerve regeneration. Journal of the Peripheral Nervous System. 2010;**15**(2):93-103. DOI: 10.1111/j.1529-8027.2010.00257.x

[48] Bigbee AJ, Hoang TX, Havton LA. At-level neuropathic pain is induced by lumbosacral ventral root avulsion injury and ameliorated by root reimplantation into the spinal cord. Experimental Neurology. 2007;**204**(1):273-282. DOI: 10.1016/j.expneurol.2006.11.003

[49] Teixeira MJ, da Paz MG da S, Bina MT, et al. Neuropathic pain after brachial plexus avulsion—Central and peripheral mechanisms. BMC Neurology. 2015;**15**:73. DOI: 10.1186/s12883-015-0329-x

[50] Yuan Q, Xie Y, So K-F, Wu W. Inflammatory response associated with axonal injury to spinal motoneurons in newborn rats. Developmental Neuroscience. 2003;**25**(1):72-78. DOI: 10.1159/000071470

[51] Carlstedt T, Cullheim S, Risling M, Ulfhake B. Nerve fibre regeneration across the PNS-CNS interface at the root-spinal cord junction. Brain Research Bulletin. 1989;**22**(1): 93-102

[52] Carlstedt T. Nerve fibre regeneration across the peripheral-central transitional zone. Journal of Anatomy. 1997;**190** (Pt 1:51-56

[53] Risling M, Sörbye K, Cullheim S. Aberrant regeneration of motor axons into the pia mater after ventral root neuroma formation. Brain Research. 1992;**570**(1-2):27-34

[54] Remahl S, Angeria M, Remahl IN, Carlstedt T, Risling M. Observations at the CNS-PNS border of ventral roots connected to a neuroma. Frontiers in Neurology. 2010;**1**:136. DOI: 10.3389/fneur.2010.00136

[55] Ohlsson M, Nieto JH, Christe KL, Havton LA. Long-term effects of a lumbosacral ventral root avulsion injury on axotomized motor neurons and avulsed ventral roots in a non-human primate model of cauda equina injury. Neuroscience. 2013;**250**:129-139. DOI: 10.1016/j.neuroscience.2013.06.054

[56] Ohlsson M, Hoang TX, Wu J, Havton LA. Glial reactions in a rodent cauda equina injury and repair model. Experimental Brain Research. 2006;**170**(1):52-60. DOI: 10.1007/s00221-005-0188-6

[57] Silver J, Miller JH. Regeneration beyond the glial scar. Nature Reviews. Neuroscience. 2004;**5**(2):146-156. DOI: 10.1038/nrn1326

[58] Yick LW, Wu W, So KF, Yip HK, Shum DK. Chondroitinase ABC promotes axonal regeneration of Clarke's neurons after spinal cord injury. Neuroreport. 2000;**11**(5):1063-1067

[59] McKeon RJ, Schreiber RC, Rudge JS, Silver J. Reduction of neurite outgrowth in a model of glial scarring following CNS injury is correlated with the expression of inhibitory molecules on reactive astrocytes. Journal of Neuroscience: The Official Journal of the Society for Neuroscience. 1991;**11**(11):3398-3411

[60] Caroni P, Schwab ME. Two membrane protein fractions from rat central myelin with inhibitory properties for neurite growth and fibroblast spreading. The Journal of Cell Biology. 1988;**106**(4):1281-1288

[61] Wang KC, Koprivica V, Kim JA, et al. Oligodendrocyte-myelin glycoprotein is a Nogo receptor ligand that inhibits neurite outgrowth. Nature. 2002;**417**(6892):941-944. DOI: 10.1038/nature00867

[62] Thanos S, Vanselow J. The effect of central and peripheral neuroglia on the regeneration of the optic nerve. Fortschritte Ophthalmologie. 1989;**86**(2):172-175

[63] Pasterkamp RJ, Verhaagen J. Emerging roles for semaphorins in neural regeneration. Brain Research. Brain Research Reviews. 2001;**35**(1):36-54

[64] Giulian D. Reactive glia as rivals in regulating neuronal survival. Glia. 1993;**7**(1):102-110. DOI: 10.1002/glia.440070116

[65] Nógrádi A, Szabó A, Pintér S, Vrbová G. Delayed riluzole treatment is able to rescue injured rat spinal motoneurons. Neuroscience. 2007;**144**(2):431-438. DOI: 10.1016/j.neuroscience.2006.09.046

[66] Wu W. Expression of nitric-oxide synthase (NOS) in injured CNS neurons as shown by NADPH diaphorase histochemistry. Experimental Neurology. 1993;**120**(2):153-159. DOI: 10.1006/exnr.1993.1050

[67] Casas C, Isus L, Herrando-Grabulosa M, et al. Network-based proteomic approaches reveal the neurodegenerative, neuroprotective and pain-related mechanisms involved after retrograde axonal damage. Scientific Reports. 2015;**5**:9185. DOI: 10.1038/srep09185

[68] Penas C, Casas C, Robert I, Forés J, Navarro X. Cytoskeletal and activity-related changes in spinal motoneurons after root avulsion. Journal of Neurotrauma. 2009;**26**(5):763-779. DOI: 10.1089/neu.2008.0661

[69] Pintér S, Gloviczki B, Szabó A, Márton G, Nógrádi A. Increased survival and reinnervation of cervical motoneurons by riluzole after avulsion of the C7 ventral root. Journal of Neurotrauma. 2010;**27**(12):2273-2282. DOI: 10.1089/neu.2010.1445

[70] Gu Y, Spasic Z, Wu W. The effects of remaining axons on motoneuron survival and NOS expression following axotomy in the adult rat. Developmental Neuroscience. 1997;**19**(3):255-259. DOI: 10.1159/000111214

[71] Wu W, Li L. Inhibition of nitric oxide synthase reduces motoneuron death due to spinal root avulsion. Neuroscience Letters. 1993;**153**(2):121-124

[72] Eggers R, Tannemaat MR, De Winter F, Malessy MJA, Verhaagen J. Clinical and neurobiological advances in promoting regeneration of the ventral root avulsion lesion. The European Journal of Neuroscience. 2016;**43**(3):318-335. DOI: 10.1111/ejn.13089

[73] Seddon HJ, Medawar PB, Smith H. Rate of regeneration of peripheral nerves in man. The Journal of Physiology. 1943;**102**(2):191-215

[74] Carlstedt T. New treatments for spinal nerve root avulsion injury. Frontiers in Neurology. 2016;**7**:135. DOI: 10.3389/fneur.2016.00135

[75] Lindå H, Risling M, Cullheim S. "Dendraxons" in regenerating motoneurons in the cat: Do dendrites generate new axons after central axotomy? Brain Research. 1985;**358**(1-2):329-333

[76] Hoang TX, Nieto JH, Havton LA. Regenerating supernumerary axons are cholinergic and emerge from both autonomic and motor neurons in the rat spinal cord. Neuroscience. 2005;**136**(2):417-423. DOI: 10.1016/j.neuroscience.2005.08.022

[77] Han L, Kan S, Yuan J. Experimental study on reimplantation of ventral root into spinal cord after brachial plexus avulsion. Zhongguo Xiu Fu Chong Jian Wai Ke Za Zhi Zhongguo Xiufu Chongjian Waike Zazhi—Chinese Journal of Reparative and Reconstructive Surgery. 2007;**21**(9):948-952

[78] Hoffmann CF, Choufoer H, Marani E, Thomeer RT. Ultrastructural study on avulsion effects of the cat cervical moto-axonal pathways in the spinal cord. Clinical Neurology and Neurosurgery. 1993;**95**(Suppl):S39-S47

[79] Kozlova EN. Strategies to repair lost sensory connections to the spinal cord. Molekuliarnaia Biologiia (Mosk). 2008;**42**(5):820-829

[80] Schlegel N, Asan E, Hofmann GO, Lang EM. Reactive changes in dorsal roots and dorsal root ganglia after C7 dorsal rhizotomy and ventral root avulsion/replantation in rabbits. Journal of Anatomy. 2007;**210**(3):336-351. DOI: 10.1111/j.1469-7580.2007.00695.x

[81] Carlstedt T. Regenerating axons form nerve terminals at astrocytes. Brain Research. 1985; **347**(1):188-191

[82] Novikov L, Novikova L, Kellerth JO. Brain-derived neurotrophic factor promotes survival and blocks nitric oxide synthase expression in adult rat spinal motoneurons after ventral root avulsion. Neuroscience Letters. 1995;**200**(1):45-48

[83] Eggers R, Tannemaat MR, Ehlert EM, Verhaagen J. A spatio-temporal analysis of motoneuron survival, axonal regeneration and neurotrophic factor expression after lumbar ventral root avulsion and implantation. Experimental Neurology. 2010;**223**(1):207-220. DOI: 10.1016/j.expneurol.2009.07.021

[84] Kemp SWP, Chiang CD, Liu EH, et al. Characterization of neuronal death and functional deficits following nerve injury during the early postnatal developmental period in rats. Developmental Neuroscience. 2015;**37**(1):66-77. DOI: 10.1159/000368769

[85] Ibrahim AG, Kirkwood PA, Raisman G, Li Y. Restoration of hand function in a rat model of repair of brachial plexus injury. Brain: A Journal of Neurology. 2009;**132**(Pt 5):1268-1276. DOI: 10.1093/brain/awp030

[86] Jivan S, Novikova LN, Wiberg M, Novikov LN. The effects of delayed nerve repair on neuronal survival and axonal regeneration after seventh cervical spinal nerve axotomy in adult rats. Experimental Brain Research. 2006;**170**(2):245-254. DOI: 10.1007/s00221-005-0207-7

[87] Lang EM, Asan E, Plesnila N, Hofmann GO, Sendtner M. Motoneuron survival after C7 nerve root avulsion and replantation in the adult rabbit: Effects of local ciliary neurotrophic factor and brain-derived neurotrophic factor application. Plastic and Reconstructive Surgery. 2005;**115**(7):2042-2050

[88] Chuang DC, Lee GW, Hashem F, Wei FC. Restoration of shoulder abduction by nerve transfer in avulsed brachial plexus injury: Evaluation of 99 patients with various nerve transfers. Plastic and Reconstructive Surgery. 1995;**96**(1):122-128

[89] Hoang TX, Pikov V, Havton LA. Functional reinnervation of the rat lower urinary tract after cauda equina injury and repair. Journal of Neuroscience: The Official Journal of the Society for Neuroscience. 2006;**26**(34):8672-8679. DOI: 10.1523/JNEUROSCI.1259-06.2006

[90] Bilgihan A, Türközkan N, Aricioğlu A, Aykol S, Cevik C, Göksel M. The effect of deferoxamine on brain lipid peroxide levels and Na-K ATPase activity following experimental subarachnoid hemorrhage. General Pharmacology. 1994;**25**(3):495-497

[91] Carlstedt T. Approaches permitting and enhancing motoneuron regeneration after spinal cord, ventral root, plexus and peripheral nerve injuries. Current Opinion in Neurology. 2000;**13**(6):683-686

[92] Carlstedt TP. Spinal nerve root injuries in brachial plexus lesions: Basic science and clinical application of new surgical strategies. A review. Microsurgery. 1995;**16**(1):13-16

[93] Chai H, Wu W, So KF, Yip HK. Survival and regeneration of motoneurons in adult rats by reimplantation of ventral root following spinal root avulsion. Neuroreport. 2000;**11**(6): 1249-1252

[94] Boyd JG, Gordon T. Neurotrophic factors and their receptors in axonal regeneration and functional recovery after peripheral nerve injury. Molecular Neurobiology. 2003;**27**(3): 277-324. DOI: 10.1385/MN:27:3:277

[95] Araújo MR, Kyrylenko S, Spejo AB, et al. Transgenic human embryonic stem cells overexpressing FGF2 stimulate neuroprotection following spinal cord ventral root avulsion. Experimental Neurology. 2017;**294**:45-57. DOI: 10.1016/j.expneurol.2017.04.009

[96] Carlstedt T, Aldskogius H, Hallin RG, Nilsson-Remahl I. Novel surgical strategies to correct neural deficits following experimental spinal nerve root lesions. Brain Research Bulletin. 1993;**30**(3-4):447-451

[97] Carlstedt T, James N, Risling M. Surgical reconstruction of spinal cord circuit provides functional return in humans. Neural Regeneration Research. 2017;**12**(12):1960-1963. DOI: 10.4103/1673-5374.221145

[98] Wang L, Yuzhou L, Yingjie Z, Jie L, Xin Z. A new rat model of neuropathic pain: Complete brachial plexus avulsion. Neuroscience Letters. 2015;**589**:52-56. DOI: 10.1016/j.neulet.2015.01.033

[99] James ND, Angéria M, Bradbury EJ, et al. Structural and functional substitution of deleted primary sensory neurons by new growth from intrinsic spinal cord nerve cells: An alternative concept in reconstruction of spinal cord circuits. Frontiers in Neurology. 2017;**8**:358. DOI: 10.3389/fneur.2017.00358

[100] Carlstedt T, Misra VP, Papadaki A, McRobbie D, Anand P. Return of spinal reflex after spinal cord surgery for brachial plexus avulsion injury. Journal of Neurosurgery. 2012; **116**(2):414-417. DOI: 10.3171/2011.7.JNS111106

[101] Gloviczki B, Török DG, Márton G, et al. Delayed spinal cord-brachial plexus reconnection after C7 ventral root avulsion: The effect of Reinnervating Motoneurons rescued by

Riluzole treatment. Journal of Neurotrauma. 2017;**34**(15):2364-2374. DOI: 10.1089/neu.2016.4754

[102] Eggers R, Hendriks WTJ, Tannemaat MR, et al. Neuroregenerative effects of lentiviral vector-mediated GDNF expression in reimplanted ventral roots. Molecular and Cellular Neurosciences. 2008;**39**(1):105-117. DOI: 10.1016/j.mcn.2008.05.018

[103] Inciong JG, Marrocco WC, Terzis JK. Efficacy of intervention strategies in a brachial plexus global avulsion model in the rat. Plastic and Reconstructive Surgery. 2000;**105**(6):2059-2071

[104] Noguchi T, Ohta S, Kakinoki R, Kaizawa Y, Matsuda S. A new cervical nerve root avulsion model using a posterior extra-vertebral approach in rats. Journal of Brachial Plexus and Peripheral Nerve Injury. 2013;**8**(1):8. DOI: 10.1186/1749-7221-8-8

[105] Wu W, Li L, Yick L-W, et al. GDNF and BDNF alter the expression of neuronal NOS, c-Jun, and p75 and prevent motoneuron death following spinal root avulsion in adult rats. Journal of Neurotrauma. 2003;**20**(6):603-612. DOI: 10.1089/089771503767168528

[106] Chin TY, Kiat SS, Faizul HG, Wu W, Abdullah JM. The effects of minocycline on spinal root avulsion injury in rat model. Malaysian Journal of Medical Sciences. 2017;**24**(1):31-39. DOI: 10.21315/mjms2017.24.1.4

[107] He J-W, Hirata K, Wang S, Kawabuchi M. Expression of nitric oxide synthase and 27-kD heat shock protein in motor neurons of ventral root-avulsed rats. Archives of Histology and Cytology. 2003;**66**(1):83-93

[108] Chang HH, Havton LA. A ventral root avulsion injury model for neurogenic underactive bladder studies. Experimental Neurology. 2016;**285**(Pt B):190-196. DOI: 10.1016/j.expneurol.2016.05.026

[109] Wu W, Han K, Li L, Schinco FP. Implantation of PNS graft inhibits the induction of neuronal nitric oxide synthase and enhances the survival of spinal motoneurons following root avulsion. Experimental Neurology. 1994;**129**(2):335-339. DOI: 10.1006/exnr.1994.1176

[110] Hoang TX, Havton LA. A single re-implanted ventral root exerts neurotropic effects over multiple spinal cord segments in the adult rat. Experimental Brain Research. 2006;**169**(2):208-217. DOI: 10.1007/s00221-005-0137-4

[111] Terzis JK, Vekris MD, Soucacos PN. Brachial plexus root avulsions. World Journal of Surgery. 2001;**25**(8):1049-1061

[112] Koliatsos VE, Clatterbuck RE, Winslow JW, Cayouette MH, Price DL. Evidence that brain-derived neurotrophic factor is a trophic factor for motor neurons in vivo. Neuron. 1993;**10**(3):359-367

[113] Henderson CE, Phillips HS, Pollock RA, et al. GDNF: A potent survival factor for motoneurons present in peripheral nerve and muscle. Science. 1994;**266**(5187):1062-1064

[114] Vejsada R, Sagot Y, Kato AC. Quantitative comparison of the transient rescue effects of neurotrophic factors on axotomized motoneurons in vivo. The European Journal of Neuroscience. 1995;**7**(1):108-115

[115] Kishino A, Ishige Y, Tatsuno T, Nakayama C, Noguchi H. BDNF prevents and reverses adult rat motor neuron degeneration and induces axonal outgrowth. Experimental Neurology. 1997;**144**(2):273-286. DOI: 10.1006/exnr.1996.6367

[116] Chu T-H, Li S-Y, Guo A, Wong W-M, Yuan Q, Wu W. Implantation of neurotrophic factor-treated sensory nerve graft enhances survival and axonal regeneration of motoneurons after spinal root avulsion. Journal of Neuropathology and Experimental Neurology. 2009;**68**(1):94-101. DOI: 10.1097/NEN.0b013e31819344a9

[117] Li L, Wu W, Lin LF, Lei M, Oppenheim RW, Houenou LJ. Rescue of adult mouse motoneurons from injury-induced cell death by glial cell line-derived neurotrophic factor. Proceedings of the National Academy of Sciences of the United States of America. 1995;**92**(21):9771-9775

[118] Noguchi T, Ohta S, Kakinoki R, et al. The neuroprotective effect of erythropoietin on spinal motor neurons after nerve root avulsion injury in rats. Restorative Neurology and Neuroscience. 2015;**33**(4):461-470. DOI: 10.3233/RNN-140481

[119] Chew DJ, Carlstedt T, Shortland PJ. The effects of minocycline or riluzole treatment on spinal root avulsion-induced pain in adult rats. Journal of Pain, the Official Journal of the American Pain Society. 2014;**15**(6):664-675. DOI: 10.1016/j.jpain.2014.03.001

[120] Kobayashi K, Imagama S, Ohgomori T, et al. Minocycline selectively inhibits M1 polarization of microglia. Cell Death & Disease. 2013;**4**:e525. DOI: 10.1038/cddis.2013.54

[121] Nógrádi A, Vrbová G. The effect of riluzole treatment in rats on the survival of injured adult and grafted embryonic motoneurons. The European Journal of Neuroscience. 2001; **13**(1):113-118

[122] Novikov LN, Novikova LN, Holmberg P, Kellerth J. Exogenous brain-derived neurotrophic factor regulates the synaptic composition of axonally lesioned and normal adult rat motoneurons. Neuroscience. 2000;**100**(1):171-181

[123] Hadaczek P, Johnston L, Forsayeth J, Bankiewicz KS. Pharmacokinetics and bioactivity of glial cell line-derived factor (GDNF) and neurturin (NTN) infused into the rat brain. Neuropharmacology. 2010;**58**(7):1114-1121. DOI: 10.1016/j.neuropharm.2010.02.002

[124] Sendtner M, Pei G, Beck M, Schweizer U, Wiese S. Developmental motoneuron cell death and neurotrophic factors. Cell and Tissue Research. 2000;**301**(1):71-84

[125] Pajenda G, Hercher D, Márton G, et al. Spatiotemporally limited BDNF and GDNF overexpression rescues motoneurons destined to die and induces elongative axon growth. Experimental Neurology. 2014;**261**:367-376. DOI: 10.1016/j.expneurol.2014.05.019

[126] Li H, Wong C, Li W, et al. Enhanced regeneration and functional recovery after spinal root avulsion by manipulation of the proteoglycan receptor PTPσ. Scientific Reports. 2015;**5**:14923. DOI: 10.1038/srep14923

[127] Chu T-H, Wu W. Neurotrophic factor treatment after spinal root avulsion injury. Central Nervous System Agents in Medicinal Chemistry. 2009;**9**(1):40-55

[128] Sakuma M, Gorski G, Sheu S-H, et al. Lack of motor recovery after prolonged denervation of the neuromuscular junction is not due to regenerative failure. The European Journal of Neuroscience. 2016;**43**(3):451-462. DOI: 10.1111/ejn.13059

[129] Sandri M, Lin J, Handschin C, et al. PGC-1alpha protects skeletal muscle from atrophy by suppressing FoxO3 action and atrophy-specific gene transcription. Proceedings of the National Academy of Sciences of the United States of America. 2006;**103**(44):16260-16265. DOI: 10.1073/pnas.0607795103

[130] Brault JJ, Jespersen JG, Goldberg AL. Peroxisome proliferator-activated receptor gamma coactivator 1alpha or 1beta overexpression inhibits muscle protein degradation, induction of ubiquitin ligases, and disuse atrophy. The Journal of Biological Chemistry. 2010; **285**(25):19460-19471. DOI: 10.1074/jbc.M110.113092

[131] Lee D, Goldberg AL. SIRT1 protein, by blocking the activities of transcription factors FoxO1 and FoxO3, inhibits muscle atrophy and promotes muscle growth. The Journal of Biological Chemistry. 2013;**288**(42):30515-30526. DOI: 10.1074/jbc.M113.489716

[132] Bahm J, El Kazzi W, Schuind F. Nerve transfers. Revue Médicale de Bruxelles. 2011;**32** (6 Suppl):S54-S57

[133] Barbour J, Yee A, Kahn LC, Mackinnon SE. Supercharged end-to-side anterior interosseous to ulnar motor nerve transfer for intrinsic musculature reinnervation. Journal of Hand Surgery. 2012;**37**(10):2150-2159. DOI: 10.1016/j.jhsa.2012.07.022

[134] Brown JM, Mackinnon SE. Nerve transfers in the forearm and hand. Hand Clinics. 2008; **24**(4):319-340. DOI: 10.1016/j.hcl.2008.08.002

[135] Korus L, Ross DC, Doherty CD, Miller TA. Nerve transfers and neurotization in peripheral nerve injury, from surgery to rehabilitation. Journal of Neurology, Neurosurgery, and Psychiatry. 2016;**87**(2):188-197. DOI: 10.1136/jnnp-2015-310420

[136] Garg R, Merrell GA, Hillstrom HJ, Wolfe SW. Comparison of nerve transfers and nerve grafting for traumatic upper plexus palsy: A systematic review and analysis. The Journal of Bone and Joint Surgery. American Volume. 2011;**93**(9):819-829. DOI: 10.2106/JBJS. I.01602

[137] Adams V. Electromyostimulation to fight atrophy and to build muscle: Facts and numbers. Journal of Cachexia, Sarcopenia and Muscle. 2018;**9**(4):631-634. DOI: 10.1002/ jcsm.12332

[138] Bueno CR de S, Pereira M, Favaretto IA, et al. Electrical stimulation attenuates morphological alterations and prevents atrophy of the denervated cranial tibial muscle. Einstein (Sao Paulo, Braz) 2017;**15**(1):71-76. DOI: 10.1590/S1679-45082017AO3808

[139] Elzinga K, Tyreman N, Ladak A, Savaryn B, Olson J, Gordon T. Brief electrical stimulation improves nerve regeneration after delayed repair in Sprague Dawley rats. Experimental Neurology. 2015;**269**:142-153. DOI: 10.1016/j.expneurol.2015.03.022

[140] Su H, Zhang W, Yang X, et al. Neural progenitor cells generate motoneuron-like cells to form functional connections with target muscles after transplantation into the musculocutaneous nerve. Cell Transplantation. 2012;**21**(12):2651-2663. DOI: 10.3727/096368912X654975

[141] Gu S, Shen Y, Xu W, et al. Application of fetal neural stem cells transplantation in delaying denervated muscle atrophy in rats with peripheral nerve injury. Microsurgery. 2010;**30**(4):266-274. DOI: 10.1002/micr.20722

[142] Ruven C, Li W, Li H, Wong W-M, Wu W. Transplantation of embryonic spinal cord derived cells helps to prevent muscle atrophy after peripheral nerve injury. International Journal of Molecular Sciences. 2017;**18**(3): 511-535. DOI: 10.3390/ijms18030511

[143] Pajer K, Nemes C, Berzsenyi S, et al. Grafted murine induced pluripotent stem cells prevent death of injured rat motoneurons otherwise destined to die. Experimental Neurology. 2015;**269**:188-201. DOI: 10.1016/j.expneurol.2015.03.031

[144] Fujimoto Y, Abematsu M, Falk A, et al. Treatment of a mouse model of spinal cord injury by transplantation of human induced pluripotent stem cell-derived long-term self-renewing neuroepithelial-like stem cells. Stem Cells (Dayt., Ohio). 2012;**30**(6):1163-1173. DOI: 10.1002/stem.1083

[145] Oda H, Ohta S, Ikeguchi R, et al. Pretreatment of nerve grafts with resveratrol improves axonal regeneration following replantation surgery for nerve root avulsion injury in rats. Restorative Neurology and Neuroscience. 2018;**36**(5):647-658. DOI: 10.3233/RNN-180844

[146] Fang X-Y, Zhang W-M, Zhang C-F, et al. Lithium accelerates functional motor recovery by improving remyelination of regenerating axons following ventral root avulsion and reimplantation. Neuroscience. 2016;**329**:213-225. DOI: 10.1016/j.neuroscience.2016.05.010

[147] Fu R, Tang Y, Ling Z-M, et al. Lithium enhances survival and regrowth of spinal motoneurons after ventral root avulsion. BMC Neuroscience. 2014;**15**:84. DOI: 10.1186/1471-2202-15-84

[148] Udina E, Ceballos D, Verdú E, Gold BG, Navarro X. Bimodal dose-dependence of FK506 on the rate of axonal regeneration in mouse peripheral nerve. Muscle & Nerve. 2002;**26**(3):348-355. DOI: 10.1002/mus.10195

[149] Labroo P, Ho S, Sant H, Shea J, Gale BK, Agarwal J. Controlled delivery of FK506 to improve nerve regeneration. Shock (Augusta, Ga.). 2016;**46**(3 Suppl 1):154-159. DOI: 10.1097/SHK.0000000000000628

[150] Labroo P, Shea J, Sant H, Gale B, Agarwal J. Effect of combining FK506 and neurotrophins on neurite branching and elongation. Muscle & Nerve. 2017;**55**(4):570-581. DOI: 10.1002/mus.25370

[151] Sugawara T, Itoh Y, Mizoi K. Immunosuppressants promote adult dorsal root regeneration into the spinal cord. Neuroreport. 1999;**10**(18):3949-3953

[152] Sun HH, Saheb-Al-Zamani M, Yan Y, Hunter DA, Mackinnon SE, Johnson PJ. Geldanamycin accelerated peripheral nerve regeneration in comparison to FK-506 in vivo. Neuroscience. 2012;**223**:114-123. DOI: 10.1016/j.neuroscience.2012.07.026

[153] Sano M. Radicicol and geldanamycin prevent neurotoxic effects of anti-cancer drugs on cultured embryonic sensory neurons. Neuropharmacology. 2001;**40**(7):947-953

[154] Romeo-Guitart D, Forés J, Navarro X, Casas C. Boosted regeneration and reduced Denervated muscle atrophy by NeuroHeal in a pre-clinical model of lumbar root avulsion with delayed Reimplantation. Scientific Reports. 2017;**7**(1):12028. DOI: 10.1038/s41598-017-11086-3

[155] Zhang C-G, Welin D, Novikov L, Kellerth J-O, Wiberg M, Hart AM. Motorneuron protection by N-acetyl-cysteine after ventral root avulsion and ventral rhizotomy. British Journal of Plastic Surgery. 2005;**58**(6):765-773. DOI: 10.1016/j.bjps.2005.04.012

[156] Scorisa JM, Zanon RG, Freria CM, de Oliveira ALR. Glatiramer acetate positively influences spinal motoneuron survival and synaptic plasticity after ventral root avulsion. Neuroscience Letters. 2009;**451**(1):34-39. DOI: 10.1016/j.neulet.2008.12.017

[157] Dyer AM, Smith A. Riluzole 5 mg/mL oral suspension: For optimized drug delivery in amyotrophic lateral sclerosis. Drug Design, Development and Therapy. 2017;**11**:59-64. DOI: 10.2147/DDDT.S123776

[158] Fukumoto T, Morinobu S, Okamoto Y, Kagaya A, Yamawaki S. Chronic lithium treatment increases the expression of brain-derived neurotrophic factor in the rat brain. Psychopharmacology. 2001;**158**(1):100-106. DOI: 10.1007/s002130100871

[159] Hoang TX, Akhavan M, Wu J, Havton LA. Minocycline protects motor but not autonomic neurons after cauda equina injury. Experimental Brain Research. 2008;**189**(1):71-77. DOI: 10.1007/s00221-008-1398-5

[160] Bowes AL, Yip PK. Modulating inflammatory cell responses to spinal cord injury: All in good time. Journal of Neurotrauma. 2014;**31**(21):1753-1766. DOI: 10.1089/neu.2014.3429

[161] Faizul HG, Wutian W, Jafri Malin A. Histological analysis of motor neuron survival and microglial inhibition after nerve root avulsion treated with nerve graft implantation and minocycline: An experimental study. Sains Malaysiana;**45**(11):1641-1648

[162] Tanaka T, Murakami K, Bando Y, Yoshida S. Minocycline reduces remyelination by suppressing ciliary neurotrophic factor expression after cuprizone-induced demyelination. Journal of Neurochemistry. 2013;**127**(2):259-270. DOI: 10.1111/jnc.12289

[163] Yune TY, Lee JY, Jung GY, et al. Minocycline alleviates death of oligodendrocytes by inhibiting pro-nerve growth factor production in microglia after spinal cord injury. Journal of Neuroscience: The Official Journal of the Society for Neuroscience. 2007; **27**(29):7751-7761. DOI: 10.1523/JNEUROSCI.1661-07.2007

[164] Pinkernelle J, Fansa H, Ebmeyer U, Keilhoff G. Prolonged minocycline treatment impairs motor neuronal survival and glial function in organotypic rat spinal cord cultures. PLoS One. 2013;**8**(8):e73422. DOI: 10.1371/journal.pone.0073422

[165] Buemi M, Cavallaro E, Floccari F, et al. The pleiotropic effects of erythropoietin in the central nervous system. Journal of Neuropathology and Experimental Neurology. 2003; **62**(3):228-236

[166] Kast RE, Altschuler EL. Consideration of acamprosate for treatment of amyotrophic lateral sclerosis. Medical Hypotheses. 2007;**69**(4):836-837. DOI: 10.1016/j.mehy.2007.01.072

[167] Man AJ, Leach JK, Bannerman P. Redirection of neurite outgrowth by coupling chondroitin sulfate proteoglycans to polymer membranes. Annals of Biomedical Engineering. 2014;**42**(6):1271-1281. DOI: 10.1007/s10439-014-0991-y

[168] Rodrigues Hell RC, Silva Costa MM, Goes AM, Oliveira ALR. Local injection of BDNF producing mesenchymal stem cells increases neuronal survival and synaptic stability following ventral root avulsion. Neurobiology of Disease. 2009;**33**(2):290-300. DOI: 10.1016/j.nbd.2008.10.017

[169] Spejo AB, Carvalho JL, Goes AM, Oliveira ALR. Neuroprotective effects of mesenchymal stem cells on spinal motoneurons following ventral root axotomy: Synapse stability and axonal regeneration. Neuroscience. 2013;**250**:715-732. DOI: 10.1016/j.neuroscience. 2013.07.043

[170] Torres-Espín A, Corona-Quintanilla DL, Forés J, et al. Neuroprotection and axonal regeneration after lumbar ventral root avulsion by re-implantation and mesenchymal stem cells transplant combined therapy. Neurother J Am Soc Exp Neurother. 2013;**10**(2): 354-368. DOI: 10.1007/s13311-013-0178-5

[171] Goméz VM, Averill S, King V, et al. Transplantation of olfactory ensheathing cells fails to promote significant axonal regeneration from dorsal roots into the rat cervical cord. Journal of Neurocytology. 2003;**32**(1):53-70

[172] Barbizan R, Castro MV, Ferreira RS, Barraviera B, Oliveira ALR. Long-term spinal ventral root reimplantation, but not bone marrow mononuclear cell treatment, positively influences ultrastructural synapse recovery and motor axonal regrowth. International Journal of Molecular Sciences. 2014;**15**(11):19535-19551. DOI: 10.3390/ijms151119535

[173] Konig N, Trolle C, Kapuralin K, et al. Murine neural crest stem cells and embryonic stem cell-derived neuron precursors survive and differentiate after transplantation in a model of dorsal root avulsion. Journal of Tissue Engineering and Regenerative Medicine. 2017; **11**(1):129-137. DOI: 10.1002/term.1893

[174] Chen L, Lu L, Meng X, Chen D, Zhang Z, Yang F. Reimplantation combined with transplantation of transgenic neural stem cells for treatment of brachial plexus root avulsion. Chinese Journal of Traumatology—Zhonghua Chuang Shang Za Zhi. 2008; **11**(5):267-273

[175] Tomita K, Hata Y, Kubo T, Fujiwara T, Yano K, Hosokawa K. Effects of the in vivo predegenerated nerve graft on early Schwann cell migration: Quantitative analysis using S100-GFP mice. Neuroscience Letters. 2009;**461**(1):36-40. DOI: 10.1016/j.neulet.2009.05.075

[176] Danielsen N, Kerns JM, Holmquist B, Zhao Q, Lundborg G, Kanje M. Pre-degenerated nerve grafts enhance regeneration by shortening the initial delay period. Brain Research. 1994;**666**(2):250-254

[177] Keilhoff G, Fansa H, Schneider W, Wolf G. In vivo predegeneration of peripheral nerves: An effective technique to obtain activated Schwann cells for nerve conduits. Journal of Neuroscience Methods. 1999;**89**(1):17-24

[178] Carbonetto S. Facilitatory and inhibitory effects of glial cells and extracellular matrix in axonal regeneration. Current Opinion in Neurobiology. 1991;**1**(3):407-413

[179] Höke A, Gordon T, Zochodne DW, Sulaiman OAR. A decline in glial cell-line-derived neurotrophic factor expression is associated with impaired regeneration after long-term Schwann cell denervation. Experimental Neurology. 2002;**173**(1):77-85. DOI: 10.1006/exnr.2001.7826

[180] de Vries J, Menovsky T, van Gulik S, Wesseling P. Histological effects of fibrin glue on nervous tissue: A safety study in rats. Surgical Neurology. 2002;**57**(6):415-422; discussion 422

[181] Kalsi P, Thom M, Choi D. Histological effects of fibrin glue and synthetic tissue glues on the spinal cord: Are they safe to use? British Journal of Neurosurgery. 2017;**31**(6):695-700. DOI: 10.1080/02688697.2017.1359491

[182] Lemaire SA, Ochoa LN, Conklin LD, et al. Nerve and conduction tissue injury caused by contact with BioGlue. The Journal of Surgical Research. 2007;**143**(2):286-293. DOI: 10.1016/j.jss.2006.10.014

[183] Barbizan R, Castro MV, Rodrigues AC, Barraviera B, Ferreira RS, Oliveira ALR. Motor recovery and synaptic preservation after ventral root avulsion and repair with a fibrin sealant derived from snake venom. PLoS One. 2013;**8**(5):e63260. DOI: 10.1371/journal.pone.0063260

[184] Vidigal de Castro M, Barbizan R, Seabra Ferreira R, Barraviera B. Leite Rodrigues de Oliveira a. Direct spinal ventral root repair following avulsion: Effectiveness of a new heterologous fibrin sealant on Motoneuron survival and regeneration. Neural Plasticity. 2016;**2932784**:2016. DOI: 10.1155/2016/2932784

[185] Wu J-C, Huang W-C, Huang M-C, et al. A novel strategy for repairing preganglionic cervical root avulsion in brachial plexus injury by sural nerve grafting. Journal of Neurosurgery. 2009;**110**(4):775-785. DOI: 10.3171/2008.8.JNS08328

[186] Lin MY, Manzano G, Gupta R. Nerve allografts and conduits in peripheral nerve repair. Hand Clinics. 2013;**29**(3):331-348. DOI: 10.1016/j.hcl.2013.04.003

[187] Magaz A, Faroni A, Gough JE, Reid AJ, Li X, Blaker JJ. Bioactive silk-based nerve guidance conduits for augmenting peripheral nerve repair. Advanced Healthcare Materials. 2018;**7**(23):e1800308. DOI: 10.1002/adhm.201800308

[188] Tang X-Q, Cai J, Nelson KD, Peng X-J, Smith GM. Functional repair after dorsal root rhizotomy using nerve conduits and neurotrophic molecules. The European Journal of Neuroscience. 2004;**20**(5):1211-1218. DOI: 10.1111/j.1460-9568.2004.03595.x

[189] Grahn PJ, Vaishya S, Knight AM, et al. Implantation of cauda equina nerve roots through a biodegradable scaffold at the conus medullaris in rat. Spine Journal: Official Journal of the North American Spine Society. 2014;**14**(9):2172-2177. DOI: 10.1016/j.spinee.2014.01.059

[190] Safa B, Buncke G. Autograft substitutes: Conduits and processed nerve allografts. Hand Clinics. 2016;**32**(2):127-140. DOI: 10.1016/j.hcl.2015.12.012

[191] Terris DJ, Toft KM, Moir M, Lum J, Wang M. Brain-derived neurotrophic factor-enriched collagen tubule as a substitute for autologous nerve grafts. Archives of Otolaryngology—Head & Neck Surgery. 2001;**127**(3):294-298

[192] Kline DG, Donner TR, Happel L, Smith B, Richter HP. Intraforaminal repair of plexus spinal nerves by a posterior approach: An experimental study. Journal of Neurosurgery. 1992;**76**(3):459-470. DOI: 10.3171/jns.1992.76.3.0459

[193] Camp SJ, Carlstedt T, Casey ATH. The lateral approach to intraspinal reimplantation of the brachial plexus: A technical note. Journal of Bone and Joint Surgery. British Volume (London). 2010;**92**(7):975-979. DOI: 10.1302/0301-620X.92B7.23778

[194] Fournier HD, Mercier P, Menei P. Repair of avulsed ventral nerve roots by direct ventral intraspinal implantation after brachial plexus injury. Hand Clinics. 2005;**21**(1):109-118. DOI: 10.1016/j.hcl.2004.09.001

[195] Fournier HD, Mercier P, Menei P. Lateral interscalenic multilevel oblique corpectomies to repair ventral root avulsions after brachial plexus injury in humans: Anatomical study and first clinical experience. Journal of Neurosurgery. 2001;**95**(2 Suppl):202-207

[196] Dubuisson AS, Kline DG, Weinshel SS. Posterior subscapular approach to the brachial plexus. Report of 102 patients. Journal of Neurosurgery. 1993;**79**(3):319-330. DOI: 10.3171/jns.1993.79.3.0319

[197] Maldonado AA, Kircher MF, Spinner RJ, Bishop AT, Shin AY. Free functioning gracilis muscle transfer with and without simultaneous intercostal nerve transfer to musculocutaneous nerve for restoration of elbow flexion after traumatic adult brachial pan-plexus injury. Journal of Hand Surgery. 2017;**42**(4):293.e1-293.e7. DOI: 10.1016/j.jhsa.2017.01.014

[198] Gu Y, Xu J, Chen L, Wang H, Hu S. Long term outcome of contralateral C7 transfer: A report of 32 cases. Chinese Medical Journal. 2002;**115**(6):866-868

[199] Wang S, Yiu H-W, Li P, Li Y, Wang H, Pan Y. Contralateral C7 nerve root transfer to neurotize the upper trunk via a modified prespinal route in repair of brachial plexus avulsion injury. Microsurgery. 2012;**32**(3):183-188. DOI: 10.1002/micr.20963

[200] Hoang TX, Havton LA. Novel repair strategies to restore bladder function following cauda equina/conus medullaris injuries. Progress in Brain Research. 2006;**152**:195-204. DOI: 10.1016/S0079-6123(05)52012-0

[201] Fournier HD, Menei P, Khalifa R, Mercier P. Ideal intraspinal implantation site for the repair of ventral root avulsion after brachial plexus injury in humans. A preliminary anatomical study. Surgical and Radiologic Anatomy. 2001;**23**(3):191-195

[202] Sáiz-Sapena N, Vanaclocha V, Insausti R, Idoate M. Dorsal root repair by means of an autologous nerve graft: Experimental study in the rat. Acta Neurochirurgica. 1997;**139**(8): 780-786

[203] Cheah M, Fawcett JW, Andrews MR. Dorsal root ganglion injection and dorsal root crush injury as a model for sensory axon regeneration. Journal of Visualized Experiments. 2017; **123**:1-7. DOI: 10.3791/55535

[204] George B, Gauthier N, Lot G. Multisegmental cervical spondylotic myelopathy and radiculopathy treated by multilevel oblique corpectomies without fusion. Neurosurgery. 1999;**44**(1):81-90

[205] null G, null L. Surgical treatment of dumbbell neurinomas of the cervical spine. Critical Reviews in Neurosurgery. 1999;**9**(3):156-160

[206] Bayerl SH, Pöhlmann F, Finger T, Prinz V, Vajkoczy P. Two-level cervical corpectomy-long-term follow-up reveals the high rate of material failure in patients, who received an anterior approach only. Neurosurgical Review. 2018; Jun:1-8. DOI: 10.1007/s10143-018-0993-6

[207] Holtzer CAJ, Marani E, van Dijk GJ, Thomeer RTWM. Repair of ventral root avulsion using autologous nerve grafts in cats. Journal of the Peripheral Nervous System. 2003; **8**(1):17-22

[208] Hoffmann CF, Thomeer RT, Marani E. Ventral root avulsions of the cat spinal cord at the brachial plexus level (cervical 7). European Journal of Morphology. 1990;**28**(2–4):418-429

[209] Amr SM, Moharram AN. Repair of brachial plexus lesions by end-to-side side-to-side grafting neurorrhaphy: Experience based on 11 cases. Microsurgery. 2005;**25**(2):126-146. DOI: 10.1002/micr.20036

Section 4

Treatment Pediatric Brachial Plexus Injuries

Chapter 5

Current Concept in the Management of Brachial Plexus Birth Palsy

Maulin Shah and Dhiren Ganjwala

Additional information is available at the end of the chapter

http://dx.doi.org/10.5772/intechopen.76109

Abstract

Most infants with brachial plexus birth palsy with signs of recovery in the first 6 weeks of life will improve spontaneously to have a normal function. However, infants who fail to recover in the first 3 months of life carry the risk of long-term disability. Panplexopathy and Horner's syndrome carry worst prognosis. Plastic neural reconstruction is indicated for the failure of return of function by 3–6 months. There is no consensus about the ideal timing of intervention, and subject is still open to debate. With microsurgical reconstruction, there is improvement in outcome in a high percentage of patients. However, any of these reconstructions is not strong enough to provide a normal function. Limited shoulder abduction and external rotation are the main elements of limitations in residual brachial plexus birth palsy children. Infants with internal contracture can be benefited with Botulinum toxin injection. Internal rotation contracture release and shoulder-rebalancing surgeries for residual brachial plexus birth palsy patients in the form of tendon transfers for congruent glenohumeral joint clearly benefit patients. Patients with noncongruent glenohumeral joint would need a derotational humeral/glenoid anteversion osteotomy. All the mentioned procedures will substantially improve but not normalize the function in children.

Keywords: obstetric palsy, natural history, microsurgery, shoulder rebalancing, bony procedure

1. Introduction

The brachial plexus is a network of peripheral nerves providing innervation to the upper extremity. Brachial plexus can be injured during labor and delivery [1]. This injury can cause stretching, rupture or avulsion of some, or all, of the cervical and first thoracic nerve roots. We prefer the term 'Brachial plexus birth palsy (BPBP)' to the more commonly used term 'obstetrical brachial palsy,' which carries implications of cause.

2. Incidence

Incidence varies from region to region and depends on the obstetrical care available in the region. The incidence of 0.42 per 1000 live births (1 in 2300) was reported in United Kingdom and Republic of Ireland [2]. Incidence is estimated to be between 1.6 and 2.6 per 1000 births [3].

3. Etiology

Shoulder dystocia is the most common cause of BPBP. The neck on the side of the anterior shoulder is stretched, and this stretch injures the brachial plexus on that side, causing a varying degree of injury. The right side is more affected as the left occipito anterior (LAO) is the most common presentation during delivery. In one study incorporating 305 infants, the author reported that 60% of patients were affected on the right side and 37% on the left side [4]. The incidence of LAO position is almost 90%, and it does not explain a higher occurrence of the left side involvement, and therefore other mechanisms like intrauterine injury to plexus is also thought of. In one study, it was observed that almost half the cases they reviewed had not shoulder dystocia, and authors concluded that it could be caused by intrauterine maladaptation and not birth trauma [5]. Another hypothesis is that the posterior shoulder can get stuck on the sacral promontory and cause injury through a stretch while the baby is in the early stage of labor before shoulder dystocia takes place [5]. There is some electrophysiological evidence to suggest that BPBP could have occurred in the intrauterine period because denervation potentials are seen in EMG performed on day 1 after delivery. This is not possible if it has occurred at the moment of delivery [6]. Interestingly, BPBP is also seen following cesarean sections [7]. Bicornuate uterus is thought to cause BPBP with phrenic palsy [8].

Macrosomia has been defined as birth weight greater than 4000–4500 g. The Royal College of Obstetricians and Gynecologists reported that BPBP is a major complication associated with macrosomia [9].

Two strategies are attempted to reduce the incidence of BPBP. The first is to consider for cesarean section when fetus is macrosomic and the second is to train obstetricians regarding the effective management of shoulder dystocia. A study to compare the incidence of BPBP from 1994 to 1998 and from 2004 to 2008 did not observe significant differences in the incidence [10], although the cesarean section rate had increased from 10.7 to 18.4%. The authors of this study concluded that despite training in the management of shoulder dystocia and a rising institutional cesarean section rate, the incidence of BPBP has remained unchanged compared with 10 years earlier.

4. Natural history

Most cases of OBPI are transient and have full recovery spontaneously. However, 10 [11]–27% [12] of children have incomplete recovery. They have lifelong functional impairment due to muscle weakness, muscle imbalance, muscle contracture, bone and joint deformities.

A cohort of 70 participants (age range 7–20 years) with different severity was assessed. Functional difference between the age of 5 years and follow-up (2–15 years) was noticed. While active shoulder and hand function remained unchanged or improved, there was a marginal reduction noted in elbow function [13].

5. Early management

5.1. Immobilization

The absolute immobilization of extremity is not advised except the child has associated clavicle or humerus fracture. Limb can be immobilized in a simple sling or a Velpeau sling for extremity fracture for a period of 2 weeks. Few mothers like to apply a pin between forearm sleeve and shirt to prevent the flaccid limb to fall on a side or get compressed while feeding the baby.

5.2. Passive range of motion exercises

Passive range of motion exercises should be started immediately to prevent the development of contractures at shoulder, elbow and wrist while waiting for brachial plexus to recover. Birch et al. suggested to carry out exercises frequently in a day, preferably before every meal [14].

5.3. Splinting

Eng et al. reported using a wrist/hand cock-up splint with thumb in opposition in patients who were developing early contractures despite regular physiotherapy [2, 15]. Shoulder external rotation splint (airplane splint) can be used to prevent internal rotation contracture at the shoulder.

5.4. Electrical stimulation

Though electrical stimulation is commonly used in practice, its efficacy is not proved.

6. Follow-up examination of newborn with BPBP

A regular monthly follow-up of patients with BPBP is recommended for various reasons in the first 3 months of life. It helps in identifying the morphologic type of injury, adaptation to different therapy protocols based on the recovery, making decision about the timing of plastic neural reconstruction of plexus and to identify and address internal rotation contractures early in its course. Neuropraxic injury recovers fully by the second month and parents can be reassured. A flaccid limb with Horner's syndrome at 3 months mounts to an indication for plastic neural reconstruction [3, 16]. Waters et al. found that children with absent biceps function at 3 months had incomplete recovery [4, 17]. Children with recovering palsy after 3 months can be followed up every two monthly. The main purpose of these visits is to see the further development of power in muscle and to identify the development of early contracture in shoulder internal contracture. Botulinum toxin injections can be considered for patients developing progressive internal rotation contracture [5, 18]. The failure to bring a cookie to the mouth without bending torso more than 45° (Cookie test) at 9 months mounts to an indication for plexus exploration and reconstruction [6, 19].

7. Investigations

7.1. Neurophysiologic investigations

7.1.1. Electromyography

The role of electromyography (EMG) in BPBP is doubtful as it frequently gives optimistic results in a severe nonresolving clinical picture. One explanation for this is the reflex-activated contraction of muscles in young children. Another explanation for this discrepancy is 'Luxury Innervation' of muscles. Until the age of 3 months, children may have polyneuronal innervation, which may give positive EMG findings in the absence of adequate nerve regeneration [7, 8, 20, 21].

7.1.2. Nerve action potentials

Although the isolated use of EMG has limitations in BPBP, according to few investigators, combining it with nerve action potentials (NAPs) may help in determining the nature and level of lesion. In selected cases, the authors have reported their ability to even differentiate axonotmesis from neurotmesis [9, 10, 14, 22].

7.2. Radiologic imaging

7.2.1. X-ray

Imaging of shoulder and upper limb can be used to diagnose the birth trauma. Chest X-ray can also give evidence of hemi diaphragm paralysis associated with C4 or phrenic nerve palsy. The diaphragm routinely lies relatively higher by two ribs level on the right side owing to liver, but in hemidiaphragm paralysis, it lies at the level of the fifth or the sixth rib.

7.2.2. Ultrasonography

Dynamic ultrasonography (USG) can help in the diagnosis of hemi diaphragm paralysis. Vathana et al. found good interobserver and intraobserver reliability in diagnosing glenohumeral deformity by ultrasound [11, 23]. Donohue et al. found measurements of glenohumeral deformity by USG reliable, but there was poor agreement between USG and magnetic resonance imaging (MRI) for diagnosing it. They questioned the use of USG as a standalone investigation for this purpose [12, 24].

7.2.3. Computed tomography scan and magnetic resonance imaging

Computed tomography (CT) myelography was considered better modality than MRI to diagnose root avulsions before a decade. Root avulsions were diagnosed based on contrast-filled meningoceles and by following the course of anterior and posterior roots from spinal cord to the respective exit foramen. But it has the disadvantage of radiation, the need of intrathecal contrast injection and the inability to reliably diagnose extra-foraminal injuries. These issues have made MRI the modality of choice for imaging brachial plexus [13, 25].

Different MRI sequences can give excellent imaging of intra-spinal as well as extra-spinal imaging of plexus. MRI can also give a clue about nerve edema, scarring and neuroma formation [14, 26].

Waters et al. reported an MRI axial image-based classification of glenohumeral deformity. It reliably measured the amount of glenoid retroversion and the percentage of humeral head anterior to mid-scapular line [15, 27]. Correlation was found between clinical parameters and MRI findings [16, 28]. The decision about surgical intervention is made on the defined congruency of glenohumeral joint on axial MRI imaging recently.

Van der Sluijis et al. found humeral head retroversion in children with BPBP after performing simultaneous axial imaging of shoulder and distal humerus [16, 28]. However, Pearl et al. recently reported that the retroversion of humeral head on the affected side is usually less compared to the normal side and discussed its merits in surgical planning [17, 29].

8. Plastic neural reconstruction

8.1. Nerve repair

8.1.1. Basis of nerve repair

Gilbert and Tassin were the first to report the comparison of conservative and surgical treatment of brachial plexus birth palsy infants in 1984 [30]. Both the groups with a similar clinical neurologic examination were compared. Sixty-three (63%) patients achieved Mallet IV shoulder function in surgical group while maximum Mallet III recovery was seen in patients with spontaneous recovery. About 27% of conservatively managed infants who showed full spontaneous recovery had gained biceps strength of MRC grade 3 by 2 months of age. End-stage improvement was incomplete in children whose biceps recovery was delayed beyond 3 months. This chapter recommended surgical intervention at 3 months, if biceps muscle has not recovered by then.

Capek et al. [31] compared the outcome of graft repair (26 patients) versus neurolysis (16 patients) of conducting neuromas. End results were found to be more promising in nerve repair group.

In patients with global injury, achieving hand function is crucial. Pondaag and Melessy have shown improved hand function after lower trunk reconstruction in about 70% of patient [32]. Gilbert and colleagues suggested that unlike adults, infants with brachial plexopathy may have the potential to regain hand function after nerve reconstructions.

8.1.2. Decision about nerve repair and its timing

It is imperative to differentiate avulsion injuries from ruptures to make microsurgical recommendations. Microsurgery is advised before 3 months of age in avulsion injuries, as spontaneous recovery cannot be expected. Ruptures can recover at different degrees, and there exists debate about the ideal indication and the time of surgery.

Gilbert and Tassin [30] considered the absence of return of biceps function by 3 months as an indication for microsurgery. Poorer global shoulder function was reported at 5 years and was associated with the further need of secondary surgeries in patients who regained biceps after 3 months. Although other researchers have followed more conservative guidelines, they have found that absent elbow flexion alone at 3 months can overestimate the poor final recovery and can lead to unneeded plexus exploration [17, 22]. They also documented that those patients who achieved biceps recovery between 4 and 6 months of age gained good global shoulder function with secondary interventions [34].

Clarke and Curtis routinely used return of biceps function at 9 months of age to determine microsurgical intervention [19, 33]. The child's ability to bring a cookie (the 'cookie test') to his or her mouth without bending the torso forward to more than 45° is a defining factor guiding treatment. Chuang et al. reported poor results of hand function while microsurgery was performed after infancy [35].

8.1.3. Technique of nerve repair

The spectrum of nerve surgery historically includes neurolysis, neuroma resection, and nerve grafting. Nerve transfers [36] and nerve conduits have led to an expansion of procedures available for nerve reconstruction. Neurolysis alone is no longer indicated in BPBP. Although few authors have reported good outcome in younger patients, direct repair of nerve endings is seldom performed after neuroma excision [37]. Nerve grafts replace the injured nerve tissue and connect the proximal and distal viable nerve endings. A number of donor grafts from the ipsilateral limb have been used; however, autologous sural nerve grafts are most commonly used [38]. Excision of neuroma with primary nerve grafting is the accepted management of nerve ruptures.

8.1.4. Outcomes of nerve repair

Clarke et al. demonstrated [39] that early improvements in neurolysis group did not sustain for a longer period of time. Patients who underwent nerve repair show significant improvement in Active Movement Scale scores at 4 years of follow-up. Erb's palsy grafting patients had improved function in seven movements, while the total palsy-grafted patients demonstrated better function in 11 of 15 movements.

Gilbert et al. have demonstrated promising long-term results in patients who have undergone nerve repair [40]. At 4 years of follow-up, 80% children with C5 C6 lesions showed good or excellent shoulder function, whereas it was 61% for children with C5–C7 lesions. Eighty-one percent of patients were graded good or excellent elbow functions at 8 years of follow-up.

After complete paralysis, the results of hand functions were quite encouraging. Although at 2 years, only 35% of children have a useful hand, after 8 years and several tendon transfers, 76% of children have a useful hand. This reflected that even lower-root avulsion should be repaired.

Birch et al. [14] published the results of nerve repair in 100 infants at mean postoperative follow-up of 85 months (30–152). They utilized Gilbert score, Mallet score and Raimondi score as outcome measures. Good results were obtained in 33% of repairs of C5, in 55% of C6, in 24% of C7 and in 57% of operations on C8 and T1. They suggested the utility of preoperative electrodiagnosis and intraoperative somatosensory-evoked potentials to detect occult intradural (pre-ganglionic) injury. Results of hand function were largely reassuring after complete paralysis. In spite of only 35% of children having a useful hand at 2 years, 76% of children enjoyed a useful hand after 8 years of follow-up and along with several tendon transfers. These results revealed the importance of repairing lower-root avulsions. Birch et al. summarized their results of nerve repairs in 100 infants after a mean follow-up of 85 months (30–152) by utilizing Gilbert score, Mallet score and Raimondi score as outcome measures. They obtained good results in 33% of C5 repairs, 55% of C6 repairs, 24% of C7 repairs and 57% of C8 and T1 repairs. They also recommended the use of preoperative electrodiagnosis and intraoperative somatosensory-evoked potentials in identifying occult intradural (pre-ganglionic) injury.

8.2. Nerve transfers

8.2.1. Basis of nerve transfers

When nerve root is avulsed from spinal cord, nerve repair is not possible. In such a case, nerve transfer connects extra brachial plexus or intraplexus functioning nerve to the nerve whose function is desired. Nerve transfer has an advantage that it permits faster reinnervation of muscle.

Various extraplexus sources like distal branch of spinal accessory nerve (SAN), intercostal nerves, hypoglossal nerve, cervical plexus, phrenic nerve and contralateral C7 root can be used for nerve transfer. In case of injury affecting C5–6 nerve roots, a fascicle from median, ulnar nerve, medial pectoral or thoracodorsal nerve can be used as donor for nerve transfer. These intraplexus nerves receive contribution predominantly from C8 and T1 roots. In global lesions, local transfers are unavailable so extraplexus nerves like intercostal nerve transfers are preferred.

The commonly used nerve transfers target to improve shoulder external rotation, abduction, elbow flexion, elbow extension and sensory function of the hand.

8.2.2. Transfer to augment external rotation of shoulder

External rotation is primarily carried out by infraspinatus muscle that is supplied by suprascapular nerve (SSN). SSN can be neurotized with SAN which can be considered an alluring extraplexal option for reviving shoulder function as it is a pure motor donor and it remains next to suprascapular nerve.

The outcomes of SAN to SSN have been published in multiple series. Nevertheless, different scoring systems were used in different papers for evaluating shoulder function; all of them implied improved shoulder functions. Only 14% of patients achieved more than 20° of active external rotation. Functional outcomes were measured by the Mallet hand to mouth and hand to neck scores. Ninety percent could reach the mouth (Mallet grade 3 or higher) and that 72% could reach the head (Mallet grade 3 or higher). These data suggest that even though there is not much improvement in external rotation, there is improvement in shoulder function. Pondaag et al. [41] determined active external rotation and functional outcome score post SAN to SSN transfers in a series of 21 patients.

Grossman [42] reported result in 26 infants who underwent SAN to SSN transfer using a nerve graft, as part of the repair of a brachial plexus birth injury. At a minimum follow-up of 2.5 years, all children had shoulder function of grade 4 or better using a modified Gilbert scale.

In another study, 54 children without return of active shoulder external rotation underwent transfer of SAN to SSN. Thirty-nine of 54 patients achieved more than 20° of active external rotation by 4 months postoperatively [25].

Terzis and Kostas [43] carried out SAN to SSN transfer in 25 children with brachial plexus birth injury. They observed improvement in abduction and external rotation component of Mallet score.

Schaakxs et al. [44] studied the results of SAN to SSN in 65 patients, the age ranging between 5 and 35 months (average 19 months) and the mean postoperative observation period of 2.5 years. They assessed their results by evaluating the recovery of passive and active external rotation with the arm in abduction and in adduction. Results were better for the external rotation with the arm in abduction compared to adduction. In 71.5% of patients, they observed active external rotation between 60 and 90°. The influence of nerve transfer on glenohumeral joint dysplasia was also assessed, and this operation has a positive influence on the glenohumeral joint.

Ruchelsman [45] reported their result of the SAN to SSN in 25 infants with brachial plexus birth injuries as part of the primary surgical reconstruction. At minimum follow-up of 24 months, the mean active external rotation was 69.6°; the mean Gilbert score was 4.1 and the mean Miami score was 7.1. These results suggest good shoulder functional outcomes.

What is the effect of age on the result? It is likely that as the denervation time increases, muscle atrophy also increases. Therefore, the delay may have negative impact on the result. Three papers analyzed this point and provided contradictory suggestions [25, 43, 45].

Satisfactory passive external rotation at shoulder is mandatory for SAN to SSN transfer. Any internal rotation contracture should be rectified surgically prior to this transfer.

8.2.3. Nerve transfer for shoulder abduction

The nerve supplying one of the heads of triceps can be transferred to the axillary nerve to improve shoulder abduction. SAN to SSN transfer aids in attaining infraspinatus and supraspinatus function. Since isolated supraspinatus is a weak abductor, deltoid activity is also required for good abduction. Neurotization of axillary nerve can help in attaining deltoid function. Each of the three heads of triceps is innervated separately by a radial nerve.

Axillary nerve passes through the quadrangular space above the teres major while the radial nerve passes through the triangular space below the teres minor. Both these nerves are in close proximity, so anastomosis is possible without nerve graft.

In a small case series of five patients, McRae reported the results of this procedure in two BPBP cases [46]. Shoulder abduction was preoperatively rated at 2 and 3 by AMS. In addition to innervations of axillary nerve, one case had SAN to SSN transfer and the other had decompression of SSN. Post SAN to SSN transfer, the respective scores were 5 and 6, illustrating antigravity shoulder abduction.

8.2.4. Nerve transfer for elbow flexion

Currently, dual transfer to innervate both biceps and brachialis is preferred for better elbow flexion strength [47]. Elbow flexion is a crucial upper limb function which can be obtained by nerve transfers to brachialis or biceps or both the muscles.

In C5–6 or C5-6-7 palsy, elbow flexion is affected; however, ulnar nerve function is normal. For such case, Oberlin transfer can be of great help for the recovery of the biceps. A fascicle of the ulnar nerve supplying the flexor carpi ulnaris muscle is cut and sutured end to end to the biceps nerve in the upper arm. Oberlin et al. [48] described this transfer in adults and Al-Qattan [49] described it for the first time for obstetric palsy in 2002.

Noaman et al. [50] reported this transfer in seven children with obstetric brachial plexus palsy. Two motor fascicles out of the ulnar nerve were transferred to the nerve to biceps. The average age at the time of operation was 16 months (range 11-24 months). The average follow-up was 19 months (range 13–30 months). Five children had biceps muscle > or = M (3) with active elbow flexion against gravity, and two children had biceps muscle <M (3).

Siqueira et al. [51] performed Oberlin's procedure in 17 infants with brachial plexus birth palsy. The mean age at the time of surgery was 12.9 months (range 4–26 months). The minimum follow-up was of 19 months. The strength of elbow flexion was measured by modified British Medical Research Council scale. Three children obtained grade 3, and 11 children had grade 4 elbow flexion power. Hand function did not deteriorate due to transfer.

Alternatively, biceps can be innervated through a fascicle of median nerve. Al-Qattan in 2014 reported their results of 10 cases of obstetric brachial plexus palsy in which median nerve to biceps nerve transfer was used [52].

Age at the time of presentation ranged from 13 to 19 months. There were seven cases of C 5–6 palsy and three cases of C5–6–7 palsy. The preoperative AMS of elbow flexion ranged from 0 to 2. At the final follow-up (1–2 years after surgery), all seven C5–6 palsy cases obtained a score of 7 out of 7 for elbow flexion. Two cases with C5–6–7 palsy had a score of 6 and 7.

8.2.5. Transfer for elbow flexion and supination

To innervate both biceps and brachialis muscles, one fascicle of both ulnar and median nerve are taken.

In a recently published paper, authors used a combined transfer in five patients and a single transfer by median or ulnar nerve fascicle in 26 patients [47]. The outcome measures were postoperative elbow flexion and supination measured with the Active Movement Scale (AMS). The mean age at surgery was 8.4 months (range 3–20 months). Patients were followed up for at least 18 months postoperatively or till they achieved full recovery of elbow flexion. Combined nerve transfer patients resulted in elbow flexion of AMS = 7 and supination of

AMS ≥ 5. Single-fascicle transfer resulted in elbow flexion of AMS ≥ 6 and supination of AMS grades 2–5. Thus, the combined transfer achieved better function.

8.2.6. Nerve transfer for elbow extension

To restore elbow extension, one possible solution is to reinnervate motor branches of radial nerve to the triceps muscle. Depending on the severity and extent of brachial plexus lesion, the radial nerve can be neurotized by means of intercostal nerves when the palsy involves the whole brachial plexus (thus, inferior roots are damaged), while in upper two or three radicular palsy, the use of fascicles of the ulnar nerve (modified Oberlin's procedure) is advisable [53].

8.2.7. Extraplexus transfer

One or two branches to the pectoralis major can be taken for the transfer so that some pectoralis major supply can be preserved and a direct repair without intervening graft can be performed to the MCN [54] or nerve to biceps [55], in the distal axilla. Intercostal nerves are an extraplexus source. They can be cut 1 cm distal to the mammary line and their stumps can be coapted directly to the MCN in the axilla.

9. Soft-tissue surgeries

Children with residual brachial plexus birth palsy frequently end up with incomplete spontaneous recovery of shoulder abduction and external rotation strength. It leads to the development of contracture of shoulder internal rotators. Progressive reduction in passive shoulder external rotation with the arm adducted is the key examination point. Studies show that the reduction of passive external rotation below neutral is associated with glenoid retroversion and humeral head posterior subluxation. Further increase in internal rotation contracture leads to flattening of humeral head and formation of biconvex glenoid, which is termed as 'false glenoid'. The aim of shoulder balancing treatment is to prevent this structural change in glenohumeral joint. Soft-tissue release to correct internal rotation contracture and tendon transfer surgeries to balance shoulder joint are possible when glenohumeral joint is congruent (Waters I–III). Once it turns non-congruent (Waters IV and V), bony procedures are offered to redirect the extremity in functional position.

9.1. Role of Botulinum toxin-A (BTX-A)

Injection of BTX-A in shoulder internal rotators temporarily denervates them while the neuronal recovery is evolving in shoulder abductors and external rotators. It is postulated that the temporary relaxation of internal rotators will help in keeping the subluxating humeral head reduced with adjunctive treatments like physiotherapy and splinting [56]. Botulinum toxin injection has also been used to treat biceps-triceps co-contraction in children with recovered palsy. Authors reported successful treatment in six patients for 18 months, where they required to inject triceps muscle twice or thrice [16, 20, 57].

http://dx.doi.org/10.5772/intechopen.76109

9.2. Role of soft-tissue release

Subscapularis is considered as the main element responsible for shoulder internal rotation contracture. Different methods of subscapularis lengthening are described in various studies with their positive and negative aspects. Gilbert reported that isolated subscapularis lengthening was enough to balance the shoulder joint in about 50% patients in their study [21, 58]. Thus, he recommended performing tendon transfer surgery in the second stage if required.

9.2.1. Open subscapularis slide from the lateral border of scapula

Subscapularis slide was introduced by Caroliz and Brahimi [58]. It involves an incision along the lateral border of scapula, approaching scapular ridge through the interval between Teres major and Teres minor. Recurrence rate was 50–70% when it was done in isolation [21, 22, 58–60]. Grossman et al. reported no recurrence when it was coupled with tendon transfer surgery [23]. Reports of ischemic necrosis of subscapularis after lateral slide pose question of safety of artery to subscapularis owing to its vicinity to the entry point for release [24, 61].

9.2.2. Minimally invasive subscapularis release

Since 2013, we have started performing subscapularis slide from the medial border of scapula through a centimeter incision placed at the junction of the upper one-third and lower two-thirds. The arm is internally rotated and the shoulder is pressed backward to make the medial border of scapula prominent (**Figure 1**). Artery forceps are advanced to make a plane between rhomboids (**Figure 2**). A small periosteal elevator is introduced in the submuscular and extra periosteal space, and subscapularis slide is done in a clockwise fashion (**Figure 3**). A larger periosteal elevator is then introduced to release stronger muscle attachments at supero-medial and inferior angle of scapula. The arm is externally rotated to achieve 90° external rotation (**Figure 4**). Conventional conjoined tendon transfer surgery was performed after minimally invasive subscapularis release (MISR). Thirty-five patients with congruent glenohumeral joint constructed the study group and were followed up for a minimum of 18 months. Improvements

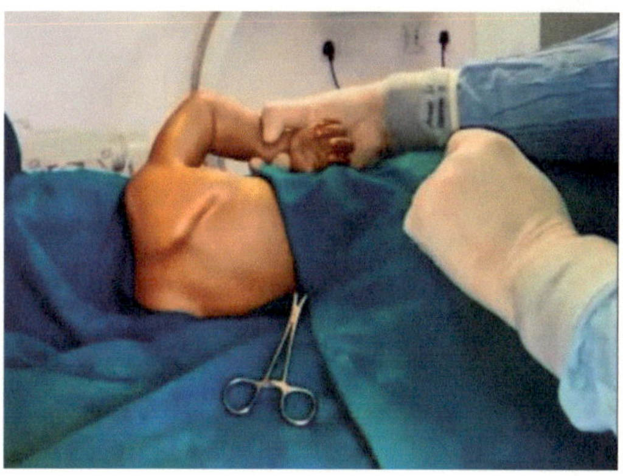

Figure 1. The arm is internally rotated to make the medial border of scapula prominent.

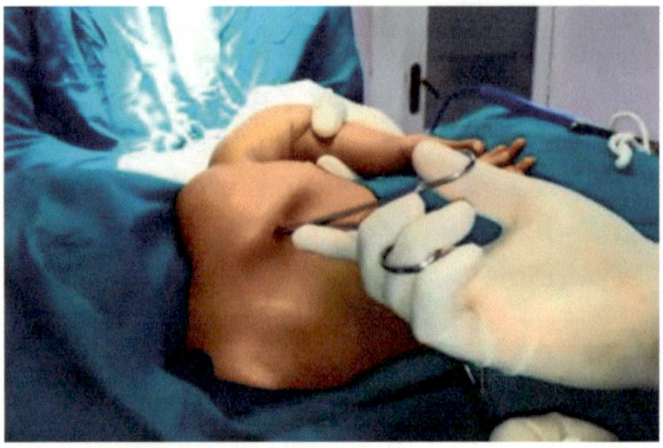

Figure 2. Rhomboids and trapezius are bluntly dissected with artery forceps.

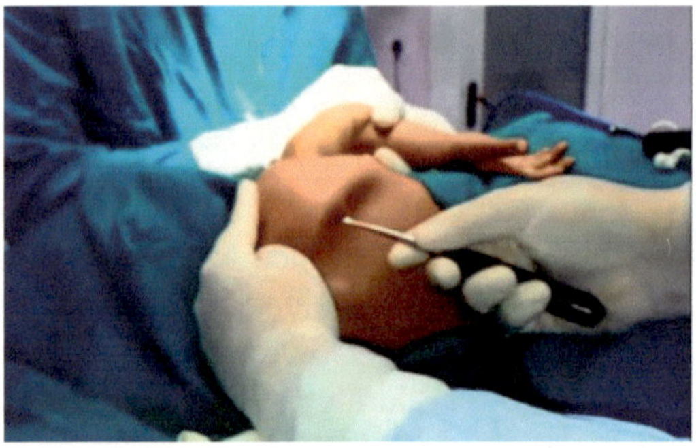

Figure 3. Periosteal elevator is inserted through the wound.

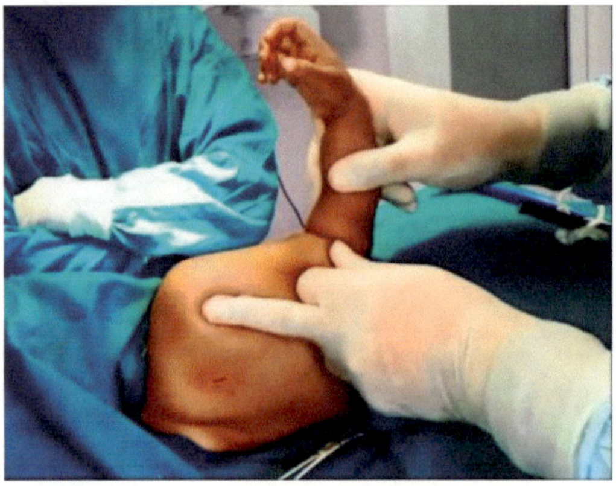

Figure 4. Shoulder is externally rotated to 90°.

in Modified Mallet scores and axial MRI parameters were comparable to the open subscapularis lengthening from insertion and arthroscopic release of subscapularis. MISR was found to have the advantage of minimal learning curve, no need of arthroscopic setup, lengthening of the muscle without weakening it and the safety of the procedure [25, 62].

9.2.3. Subscapularis lengthening from insertion

Partial lengthening or z-plasty of subscapularis through anterior incision has been described. Van der Juis reported that excessive release of muscle from insertion leads to external rotation contracture and anterior shoulder instability. A subset of patients in their series required secondary internal rotation osteotomy [26, 63].

9.2.4. Arthroscopic subscapularis and soft-tissue release

Pearl et al. reported results of arthroscopic soft-tissue release with the help of a 2.7-mm arthroscope [64]. Children younger than 4 years received the release of tendinous part of subscapularis and capsulo-ligamentous structures, while the older children also had lattissimus dorsi transfer. Four of the 19 patients who received only soft-tissue release required tendon transfer surgery later. Three out of these four children had pseudoglenoid on preoperative imaging. The major issue related to arthroscopic release was the loss of internal rotation range [27].

9.3. Tendon transfer surgery to improve external rotation

L'Episcopo primarily reported muscle transfers for residual brachial plexus palsy patients in 1934 [28]. It was sub-sequentially altered by Hoffer [65]. Latissimus dorsi and teres major transfer to rotator cuff along with the release of pectoralis major has demonstrated enhanced active external rotation of 45° and abduction of 64° at 2–8 years of follow-up [66].

Waters et al. reported halting of glenohumeral deformity from progression after these transfers with extraarticular soft-tissue release [67]. Greenhill et al. compared a combined conjoined tendon transfer to isolated Teres major transfer. They found similar improvements in external rotation in both transfers but the incidence of limited midline function was found more in combined transfers. They recommended isolated Teres major transfer where preoperative midline function was in question [68].

9.4. Tendon transfer surgery to improve shoulder abduction

Cheung et al. proposed the theory of co-contraction between agonist and antagonist muscles while they are recovering, leading to the restriction of particular movement across the shoulder joint. They advocated lateral trans-positioning of clavicular part of pectoralis major along with Teres major transfer to infraspinatus. The authors reported the average gain in abduction of 77° in their cohort [69, 70]. Improvement in abduction has been reported in patients where conjoined teres major and lattissimus dorsi tendons were transferred to infraspinatus without pectoralis major trans-positioning [31].

10. Bony procedures

10.1. Humeral rotational osteotomy

Many late presenting cases may have developed glenohumeral dysplasia at the time of presentation. For such situations, humeral derotation osteotomy is one option to improve the function. Humeral derotation osteotomy does not improve the range of motion (ROM) of glenohumeral motion but reorients the arc of shoulder rotation into a more functional range which improves the function.

10.1.1. Indications of humerus osteotomy

Moderate-to-severe glenohumeral deformity (Waters Grades III–V) has restricted external rotation and abduction.

10.1.2. Surgical technique

Through a delto-pectoral approach, proximal humerus is exposed. Osteotomy is carried out just proximal to the insertion of deltoid. Distal fragment is rotated externally and is held firmly by the bone holding forceps. Before final fixation, it is confirmed that the hand can be easily placed to the mouth, occiput, perineum and midline in an effort to avoid overcorrection. This important step prevents overcorrection as well as under-correction.

10.1.3. Results

Kirkos and Papadopoulos [71] reported the results for 22 patients who underwent humerus derotation osteotomy. The authors have shown improvement in shoulder abduction of 27° and external rotation of 25° at a mean follow-up of 14 years (ranges from 2 to 31 years). An increase in forearm supination was also noted following improvement in shoulder external rotation.

Al-Qattan [72] also reported the results in a series of 15 children. At an average follow-up of 3 years, the patients demonstrated improvement in the mean modified Mallet score for hand-to-neck motion. It increased from 2.2 to 4 points.

Waters and Bae [73] used this operation in 28 patients. Osteotomy was fixed stably with internal fixation. All patients demonstrated improvements in shoulder function postoperatively, as evidenced by improved aggregate Mallet scores. The mean aggregate Mallet classification score improved from 13 points preoperatively to 18 points postoperatively.

10.2. Glenoid anteversion osteotomy

Hopyan and colleagues combined glenoid neck osteotomy with soft-tissue rebalancing surgeries [74]. The purpose of their study was to see whether glenoid reorientation converts a shoulder joint from one where tendon transfer and soft-tissue release cannot restore the active motion to the one where it can. They found improved Mallet scores for global external rotation and hand-to-neck movements. Waters schema was found improved from average of 4.3 preoperatively to 1.6 postoperatively. This novel technique was proposed as an alternative to humeral derotation osteotomy.

http://dx.doi.org/10.5772/intechopen.76109

11. Conclusion

Results of BPBP have improved substantially by various advances that have taken place in the last four decades. We can achieve functional improvement in a majority of cases, but still most cases do not achieve a full functional recovery. Improvement in the surgical technique will lead to better outcome. On the other hand, efforts to prevent this condition will also yield greater benefit.

Author details

Maulin Shah[1]* and Dhiren Ganjwala[2]

*Address all correspondence to: maulinmshah@gmail.com

1 Orthokids Hospital, Ahmedabad, India

2 Ganjwala Hospital, Ahmedabad, India

References

[1] Tan KL. Brachial palsy. The Journal of Obstetrics and Gynaecology of the British Commonwealth. 1973;**80**(1):60-62

[2] Evans-Jones G, Kay SP, Weindling AM, Cranny G, Ward A, Bradshaw A, et al. Congenital brachial palsy: Incidence, causes, and outcome in the United Kingdom and Republic of Ireland. Archives of Disease in Childhood. Fetal and Neonatal Edition. 2003 May;**88**(3):F185-F189

[3] Coroneos CJ, Voineskos SH, Coroneos MK, Alolabi N, Goekjian SR, Willoughby LI, et al. Primary nerve repair for obstetrical brachial plexus injury: A meta-analysis. Plastic and Reconstructive Surgery. 2015 Oct;**136**(4):765-779

[4] Thatte MR, Mehta R. Obstetric brachial plexus injury. Indian Journal of Plastic Surgery. 2011 Sep;**44**(3):380-389

[5] Jennett RJ, Tarby TJ, Kreinick CJ. Brachial plexus palsy: An old problem revisited. American Journal of Obstetrics and Gynecology. 1992 Jun;**166**(6 Pt 1):1673-1676; discussion 6-7

[6] Alfonso DT. Causes of neonatal brachial plexus palsy. Bulletin of the NYU Hospital for Joint Diseases. 2011;**69**(1):11-16

[7] Gherman RB, Goodwin TM, Ouzounian JG, Miller DA, Paul RH. Brachial plexus palsy associated with cesarean section: An in utero injury? American Journal of Obstetrics and Gynecology. 1997 Nov;**177**(5):1162-1164

[8] Dunn DW, Engle WA. Brachial plexus palsy: Intrauterine onset. Pediatric Neurology. 1985 Nov-Dec;**1**(6):367-369

[9] Chauhan SP, Gherman R, Hendrix NW, Bingham JM, Hayes E. Shoulder dystocia: Comparison of the ACOG practice bulletin with another national guideline. American Journal of Perinatology. 2010;**27**(02):129-136

[10] Walsh JM, Kandamany N, Ni Shuibhne N, Power H, Murphy JF, O'Herlihy C. Neonatal brachial plexus injury: Comparison of incidence and antecedents between 2 decades. American Journal of Obstetrics and Gynecology. 2011 Apr;**204**(4):324 e1-324 e6

[11] Walle T, Hartikainen-Sorri AL. Obstetric shoulder injury. Associated risk factors, prediction and prognosis. Acta Obstetricia et Gynecologica Scandinavica. 1993 Aug;**72**(6):450-454

[12] Jackson ST, Hoffer MM, Parrish N. Brachial-plexus palsy in the newborn. The Journal of Bone and Joint Surgery. American Volume. 1988 Sep;**70**(8):1217-1220

[13] Strombeck C, Krumlinde-Sundholm L, Remahl S, Sejersen T. Long-term follow-up of children with obstetric brachial plexus palsy I: Functional aspects. Developmental Medicine and Child Neurology. 2007 Mar;**49**(3):198-203

[14] Birch R, Ahad N, Kono H, Smith S. Repair of obstetric brachial plexus palsy: Results in 100 children. Journal of Bone and Joint Surgery. British Volume (London). 2005 Aug;**87**(8):1089-1095

[15] Eng GD, Binder H, Getson P, O'Donnell R. Obstetrical brachial plexus palsy (OBPP) outcome with conservative management. Muscle & Nerve. 1996 Jul;**19**(7):884-891

[16] Gilbert A. Long-term evaluation of brachial plexus surgery in obstetrical palsy. Hand Clinics. 1995 Nov;**11**(4):583-594; discussion 94-5

[17] Waters PM. Comparison of the natural history, the outcome of microsurgical repair, and the outcome of operative reconstruction in brachial plexus birth palsy. The Journal of Bone and Joint Surgery. American Volume. 1999 May;**81**(5):649-659

[18] Ezaki M, Malungpaishrope K, Harrison RJ, Mills JK, Oishi SN, Delgado M, et al. Onabotulinum toxinA injection as an adjunct in the treatment of posterior shoulder subluxation in neonatal brachial plexus palsy. The Journal of Bone and Joint Surgery. American Volume. 2010 Sep 15;**92**(12):2171-2177

[19] Clarke HM, Curtis CG. An approach to obstetrical brachial plexus injuries. Hand Clinics. 1995 Nov;**11**(4):563-580; discussion 80-1

[20] Hesselmans LF, Jennekens FG, Van den Oord CJ, Veldman H, Vincent A. Development of innervation of skeletal muscle fibers in man: Relation to acetylcholine receptors. The Anatomical Record. 1993 Jul;**236**(3):553-562

[21] Ijkema-Paassen J, Gramsbergen A. Polyneural innervation in the psoas muscle of the developing rat. Muscle & Nerve. 1998 Aug;**21**(8):1058-1063

[22] Smith NC, Rowan P, Benson LJ, Ezaki M, Carter PR. Neonatal brachial plexus palsy. Outcome of absent biceps function at three months of age. The Journal of Bone and Joint Surgery. American Volume. 2004 Oct;**86-A**(10):2163-2170

[23] Vathana T, Rust S, Mills J, Wilkes D, Browne R, Carter PR, et al. Intraobserver and interobserver reliability of two ultrasound measures of humeral head position in infants with neonatal brachial plexus palsy. The Journal of Bone and Joint Surgery. American Volume. 2007 Aug;**89**(8):1710-1715

[24] Donohue KW, Little KJ, Gaughan JP, Kozin SH, Norton BD, Zlotolow DA. Comparison of ultrasound and MRI for the diagnosis of glenohumeral dysplasia in brachial plexus birth palsy. The Journal of Bone and Joint Surgery. American Volume. 2017 Jan;**99**(2):123-132

[25] van Ouwerkerk WJ, Uitdehaag BM, Strijers RL, Frans N, Holl K, Fellner FA, et al. Accessory nerve to suprascapular nerve transfer to restore shoulder exorotation in otherwise spontaneously recovered obstetric brachial plexus lesions. Neurosurgery. 2006 Oct;**59**(4):858-867; discussion 67-9

[26] Martin Noguerol T, Barousse R, Socolovsky M, Luna A. Quantitative magnetic resonance (MR) neurography for evaluation of peripheral nerves and plexus injuries. Quantitative Imaging in Medicine and Surgery. 2017 Aug;**7**(4):398-421

[27] Waters PM, Smith GR, Jaramillo D. Glenohumeral deformity secondary to brachial plexus birth palsy. The Journal of Bone and Joint Surgery. American Volume. 1998 May; **80**(5):668-677

[28] van der Sluijs JA, van Ouwerkerk WJ, de Gast A, Wuisman P, Nollet F, Manoliu RA. Retroversion of the humeral head in children with an obstetric brachial plexus lesion. Journal of Bone and Joint Surgery. British Volume (London). 2002 May;**84**(4):583-587

[29] Pearl ML, Batech M, van de Bunt F. Humeral retroversion in children with shoulder internal rotation contractures secondary to upper-trunk neonatal brachial plexus palsy. The Journal of Bone and Joint Surgery. American Volume. 2016 Dec;**98**(23):1988-1995

[30] Gilbert A, Tassin JL. Surgical repair of the brachial plexus in obstetric paralysis. Chirurgie. 1984;**110**(1):70-75

[31] Capek L, Clarke HM, Curtis CG. Neuroma-in-continuity resection: Early outcome in obstetrical brachial plexus palsy. Plastic and Reconstructive Surgery. 1998 Oct;**102**(5): 1555-1562; discussion 63-4

[32] Pondaag W, Malessy MJ. Recovery of hand function following nerve grafting and transfer in obstetric brachial plexus lesions. Journal of Neurosurgery. 2006 Jul;**105**(1 Suppl): 33-40

[33] Bain JR, Dematteo C, Gjertsen D, Hollenberg RD. Navigating the gray zone: A guideline for surgical decision making in obstetrical brachial plexus injuries. Journal of Neurosurgery. Pediatrics. 2009 Mar;**3**(3):173-180

[34] Al-Qattan MM. The outcome of Erb's palsy when the decision to operate is made at 4 months of age. Plastic and Reconstructive Surgery. 2000 Dec;**106**(7):1461-1465

[35] Chuang DC, Mardini S, Ma HS. Surgical strategy for infant obstetrical brachial plexus palsy: Experiences at Chang Gung Memorial Hospital. Plastic and Reconstructive Surgery. 2005 Jul;**116**(1):132-142; discussion 43-4

[36] El-Gammal TA, Fathi NA. Outcomes of surgical treatment of brachial plexus injuries using nerve grafting and nerve transfers. Journal of Reconstructive Microsurgery. 2002 Jan;**18**(1):7-15

[37] Kirjavainen M, Remes V, Peltonen J, Kinnunen P, Poyhia T, Telaranta T, et al. Long-term results of surgery for brachial plexus birth palsy. The Journal of Bone and Joint Surgery. American Volume. 2007 Jan;**89**(1):18-26

[38] Midha R. Nerve transfers for severe brachial plexus injuries: A review. Neurosurgical Focus. 2004 May;**16**(5):E5

[39] Lin JC, Schwentker-Colizza A, Curtis CG, Clarke HM. Final results of grafting versus neurolysis in obstetrical brachial plexus palsy. Plastic and Reconstructive Surgery. 2009 Mar;**123**(3):939-948

[40] Gilbert A, Pivato G, Kheiralla T. Long-term results of primary repair of brachial plexus lesions in children. Microsurgery. 2006;**26**(4):334-342

[41] Pondaag W, de Boer R, van Wijlen-Hempel MS, Hofstede-Buitenhuis SM, Malessy MJ. External rotation as a result of suprascapular nerve neurotization in obstetric brachial plexus lesions. Neurosurgery. 2005 Sep;**57**(3):530-537; discussion 7

[42] Grossman JA, Di Taranto P, Alfonso D, Ramos LE, Price AE. Shoulder function following partial spinal accessory nerve transfer for brachial plexus birth injury. Journal of Plastic, Reconstructive & Aesthetic Surgery. 2006;**59**(4):373-375

[43] Terzis JK, Kostas I. Outcomes with suprascapular nerve reconstruction in obstetrical brachial plexus patients. Plastic and Reconstructive Surgery. 2008 Apr;**121**(4):1267-1278

[44] Schaakxs D, Bahm J, Sellhaus B, Weis J. Clinical and neuropathological study about the neurotization of the suprascapular nerve in obstetric brachial plexus lesions. Journal of Brachial Plexus and Peripheral Nerve Injury. 2009 Sep;**4**:15

[45] Ruchelsman DE, Ramos LE, Alfonso I, Price AE, Grossman A, Grossman JA. Outcome following spinal accessory to suprascapular (spinoscapular) nerve transfer in infants with brachial plexus birth injuries. Hand (N Y). 2010 Jun;**5**(2):190-194

[46] McRae MC, Borschel GH. Transfer of triceps motor branches of the radial nerve to the axillary nerve with or without other nerve transfers provides antigravity shoulder abduction in pediatric brachial plexus injury. Hand (N Y). 2012 Jun;**7**(2):186-190

[47] Little KJ, Zlotolow DA, Soldado F, Cornwall R, Kozin SH. Early functional recovery of elbow flexion and supination following median and/or ulnar nerve fascicle transfer in upper neonatal brachial plexus palsy. The Journal of Bone and Joint Surgery. American Volume. 2014 Feb;**96**(3):215-221

[48] Oberlin C, Beal D, Leechavengvongs S, Salon A, Dauge MC, Sarcy JJ. Nerve transfer to biceps muscle using a part of ulnar nerve for C5-C6 avulsion of the brachial plexus: Anatomical study and report of four cases. Journal of Hand Surgery American Society for Surgery of the Hand. 1994 Mar;**19**(2):232-237

[49] Al-Qattan MM. Oberlin's ulnar nerve transfer to the biceps nerve in Erb's birth palsy. Plastic and Reconstructive Surgery. 2002 Jan;**109**(1):405-407

[50] Noaman HH, Shiha AE, Bahm J. Oberlin's ulnar nerve transfer to the biceps motor nerve in obstetric brachial plexus palsy: Indications, and good and bad results. Microsurgery. 2004;**24**(3):182-187

[51] Siqueira MG, Socolovsky M, Heise CO, Martins RS, Di Masi G. Efficacy and safety of Oberlin's procedure in the treatment of brachial plexus birth palsy. Neurosurgery. 2012 Dec;**71**(6):1156-1160; discussion 61

[52] Al-Qattan MM, Al-Kharfy TM. Median nerve to biceps nerve transfer to restore elbow flexion in obstetric brachial plexus palsy. BioMed Research International. 2014;**2014**:854084

[53] Senes FM, Catena N, Dapelo E, Senes J. Nerve transfer for elbow extension in obstetrical brachial plexus palsy. Annals of the Academy of Medicine, Singapore. 2016 May;**45**(5): 221-224

[54] Blaauw G, Slooff AC. Transfer of pectoral nerves to the musculocutaneous nerve in obstetric upper brachial plexus palsy. Neurosurgery. 2003 Aug;**53**(2):338-341; discussion 41-2

[55] Pondaag W, Malessy MJ. Intercostal and pectoral nerve transfers to re-innervate the biceps muscle in obstetric brachial plexus lesions. The Journal of Hand Surgery, European Volume. 2014 Jul;**39**(6):647-652

[56] Maulin S. Botulinum toxin injection for shoulder joint imbalance in infants with residual obstetric brachial plexus palsy; does it change the natural history? Pediatric Orthopaedics Society of India Conference; Bangalore; 2016.

[57] Heise CO, Goncalves LR, Barbosa ER, Gherpelli JL. Botulinum toxin for treatment of cocontractions related to obstetrical brachial plexopathy. Arquivos de Neuro-Psiquiatria. 2005 Sep;**63**(3A):588-591

[58] Carlioz H, Brahimi L. Place of internal disinsertion of the subscapularis muscle in the treatment of obstetric paralysis of the upper limb in children. Annales de Chirurgie Infantile. 1971 Mar-Apr;**12**(2):159-167

[59] Newman CJ, Morrison L, Lynch B, Hynes D. Outcome of subscapularis muscle release for shoulder contracture secondary to brachial plexus palsy at birth. Journal of Pediatric Orthopedics. 2006 Sep-Oct;**26**(5):647-651

[60] Immerman I, Valencia H, DiTaranto P, DelSole EM, Glait S, Price AE, et al. Subscapularis slide correction of the shoulder internal rotation contracture after brachial plexus birth injury: Technique and outcomes. Techniques in Hand & Upper Extremity Surgery. 2013 Mar;**17**(1):52-56

[61] Chen L, Gu Y, Xu J. Operative treatment of medial rotation contracture of the shoulder caused by obstetric brachial plexus palsy. Chinese Journal of Traumatology. 2000 Feb;**3**(1):13-17

[62] Maulin S. Minimally Invasive Subscapularis Release: A Novel Technique & Early Results. In: Pediatric Orthopaedics Society of India Conference; Nagpur: 2017

[63] van der Sluijs JA, van Ouwerkerk WJ, de Gast A, Nollet F, Winters H, Wuisman PI. Treatment of internal rotation contracture of the shoulder in obstetric brachial plexus lesions by subscapular tendon lengthening and open reduction: Early results and complications. Journal of Pediatric Orthopaedics. Part B. 2004 May;**13**(3):218-224

[64] Pearl ML, Edgerton BW, Kazimiroff PA, Burchette RJ, Wong K. Arthroscopic release and latissimus dorsi transfer for shoulder internal rotation contractures and glenohumeral deformity secondary to brachial plexus birth palsy. The Journal of Bone and Joint Surgery. American Volume. 2006 Mar;**88**(3):564-574

[65] Hoffer MM, Wickenden R, Roper B. Brachial plexus birth palsies. Results of tendon transfers to the rotator cuff. The Journal of Bone and Joint Surgery. American Volume. 1978 Jul;**60**(5):691-695

[66] Phipps GJ, Hoffer MM. Latissimus dorsi and teres major transfer to rotator cuff for Erb's palsy. Journal of Shoulder and Elbow Surgery. 1995 Mar-Apr;**4**(2):124-129

[67] Waters PM, Bae DS. Effect of tendon transfers and extra-articular soft-tissue balancing on glenohumeral development in brachial plexus birth palsy. The Journal of Bone and Joint Surgery. American Volume. 2005 Feb;**87**(2):320-325

[68] Greenhill DA, Smith WR, Ramsey FV, Kozin SH, Zlotolow DA. Double versus single tendon transfers to improve shoulder function in brachial plexus birth palsy. Journal of Pediatric Orthopedics. 2017 Mar

[69] Chuang DC, Ma HS, Wei FC. A new evaluation system to predict the sequelae of late obstetric brachial plexus palsy. Plastic and Reconstructive Surgery. 1998 Mar;**101**(3):673-685

[70] Chuang DC, Ma HS, Wei FC. A new strategy of muscle transposition for treatment of shoulder deformity caused by obstetric brachial plexus palsy. Plastic and Reconstructive Surgery. 1998 Mar;**101**(3):686-694

[71] Kirkos JM, Papadopoulos IA. Late treatment of brachial plexus palsy secondary to birth injuries: Rotational osteotomy of the proximal part of the humerus. The Journal of Bone and Joint Surgery. American Volume. 1998 Oct;**80**(10):1477-1483

[72] Al-Qattan MM. Rotation osteotomy of the humerus for Erb's palsy in children with humeral head deformity. Journal of Hand Surgery American Society for Surgery of the Hand. 2002 May;**27**(3):479-483

[73] Waters PM, Bae DS. The effect of derotational humeral osteotomy on global shoulder function in brachial plexus birth palsy. The Journal of Bone and Joint Surgery. American Volume. 2006 May;**88**(5):1035-1042

[74] Dodwell E, O'Callaghan J, Anthony A, Jellicoe P, Shah M, Curtis C, et al. Combined glenoid anteversion osteotomy and tendon transfers for brachial plexus birth palsy: Early outcomes. The Journal of Bone and Joint Surgery. American Volume. 2012 Dec;**94**(23):2145-2152

Section 5

Treatment of Brachial Plexus Long Term Consequences

Chapter 6

Treatment of Neuropathic Pain in Brachial Plexus Injuries

Nieves Saiz-Sapena,
Vicente Vanaclocha-Vanaclocha,
José María Ortiz-Criado, L. Vanaclocha and
Nieves Vanaclocha

Additional information is available at the end of the chapter

http://dx.doi.org/10.5772/intechopen.82084

Abstract

Brachial plexus injuries are commonly followed by chronic pain, mostly with neuropathic characteristics. This is due to peripheral nerve lesions, particularly nerve root avulsions, as well as upper limb amputations, and complex regional pain syndrome (CRPS). The differential diagnosis between CRPS and neuropathic pain is essential as the treatment is different for each of them. Medical treatments are the first step, but for refractory cases there are two main types of surgical alternatives: ablative techniques and neuromodulation. The first group involves destruction of the posterior horn deafferented neurons and usually provides a better pain control but has a 10% complication rate. The second group provides pain control with function preservation but with limited effectiveness. Each case has to be thoroughly evaluated to apply the treatment modality best suited for it.

Keywords: brachial plexus injury, brachial plexus avulsion, chronic pain, neuropathic pain, deafferentation pain, phantom pain, pulsed radiofrequency, peripheral nerve stimulation, neuromodulation, DREZ-otomy

1. Introduction

Brachial plexus injuries are associated not only with motor and sensory functional impairment [1] but also with chronic pain in the affected upper limb [2–7]. Most of these injuries are due to motor vehicle accidents, particularly motorbikes [1, 5], but a few of them can occur due to iatrogenia [8–16], particularly during lymph node biopsy [17, 18] or treatment of some malignancies [19].

The *pain* is chronic [20], persistent [7], constant [21], burning [22] and throbbing [17], with paroxysmal discharges [3, 6, 23], particularly upon gentle rubbing the affected area [4].

The *pain is distributed* in the distal areas of the upper limb, covering several dermatomes, mostly the caudal ones [24] and particularly the hand [5, 17, 23, 25]. The paroxysmal pain is felt in the arm [26]. Allodynia, hypersensitivity and electric-like discharges are present at the border between the normal and affected dermatomes [17, 26–29], particularly between T_1 and T_2 at the posterior aspect of the elbow [26].

The *pain severity* correlates with the magnitude of the brachial plexus injury [2, 3] and to the number of avulsed nerve roots [2–4, 21, 26, 30–33], particularly when the lower roots are affected [24, 34, 35]. Nevertheless, Bertelli et al. [21] found that in isolated C_8 and T_1 nerve root avulsions, there was no pain at all.

The *pain* does not *appear* immediately after the injury but a few days later [24] and no longer than 3 months after it [5, 6, 24, 26, 35, 36].

The *neuropathic pain can be associated with* phantom [37] or stump pain [38] in case of upper limb amputation, or to complex regional pain syndrome (CRPS) [6], inducing a complex pain condition rather difficult to control [19, 30, 31].

Self-mutilation has been described in 5–29% of obstetric brachial plexus injury cases [39, 40].

The *quality of life* is seriously impaired with sleep disorders, family troubles, unemployment, chronic depression and social withdrawal [2, 5, 6, 17, 21, 41–44]. Additionally, the chronic pain is a further hindrance to comply with a good rehabilitation programme, impairing a possible functional recovery [6, 45, 46]. Among all the disabilities induced by the brachial plexus injury, the pain has been found to be the symptom that most negatively affects the quality of life [47].

Treatment of this chronic pain can be troublesome, as the response to the different treatment modalities is poor and not all of them allow preservation of the remaining upper limb function [2, 5, 48].

2. Incidence

Although 50–82.7% of brachial plexus injuries suffer from chronic pain [2, 3, 5, 6, 17, 35, 49–51], it is severe in 41% of them [32]. The incidence and severity are higher in nerve root avulsions [2–4, 7, 21, 30, 33], especially when all the roots are avulsed [2, 17, 21]. Overtime there is a spontaneous progressive improvement, so just after the injury 90% of patients suffer from pain but affects only 30% of them 3 years later [35, 36, 49].

Predisposing factors: the strongest is alcohol abuse [17], but smoking [6, 17], other coexistent pain conditions [6], like psychiatric co-morbidities [6, 17], using a sling [5] and the marital status (both married or divorced versus being single) also increase the pain incidence [5]. A longer time using a sling increases the chance of chronic pain because limb movement restriction has a negative impact on recovery [5].

Brachial plexus injuries may also be accompanied by partial or complete traumatic upper limb amputation. About *50–85%* of these *amputees* will suffer from *chronic pain* [52, 53] particularly in more proximal amputations [53]. This pain usually starts 1 month postamputation [53], and in 54–87% of them, it is followed by *phantom limb pain* [37, 53, 54]. This kind of pain is felt also in extensive nerve root avulsions, particularly when all of them are affected [55].

CRPS is present in 21% of brachial plexus injuries [6], and once it starts it is usually lifelong unless treated [35].

3. Pathophysiology

The neuropathic pain is induced by an injury to the somatosensory pathways [56, 57] like a brachial plexus injury, an upper limb amputation or both of them simultaneously [2, 7, 58].

The peripheral nerve injury induces deafferentation [2] and damage to the C nerve fibres [59]. The dorsal horn neurons devoid of their peripheral sensorial input start to fire spontaneously and erratically [60–64], stimulating pain sensation in the higher central nervous system levels [65, 66]. In experimental studies it has been found that the spinal cord microglia and astrocytes are activated at the injury site [67] and help to maintain the neuropathic pain [68–72]. Higher levels like the thalamus and the motor cortex also undergo the same process by which deafferented neurons create new synapses and reorganize and start firing in abnormal patterns [7, 73–77]. Descending pathways modulate the neuropathic pain [78] creating new circuits that induce and maintain it [79–81]. The brain and spinal cord neuronal reorganization leads to an increased sensitivity to otherwise normal stimuli, lowering the threshold required to feel the sensation as pain and inducing secondary hyperalgesia and allodynia [4, 82]. It also explains why the pain often extends beyond the denervated area [26, 33] and why it manifests at the border areas between the partially denervated and normal dermatomes [17, 27].

As mentioned above the pain seen after brachial plexus injury has two distinct patterns: paroxysmal and continuous. The first one is thought to originate from the deafferented posterior spinal horn neurons [60, 83], while the second one comes from the thalamus [74, 84]. In the phantom limb pain, the brain cortex undergoes a functional reorganization in response to the chronic pain [40, 85, 86].

Some have suggested that the neuropathic pain after brachial plexus avulsion is generated not by the avulsed nerve roots but by the remaining ones [67] that are also injured, although not so severely [34]. Although this might be true in some cases, it does not explain why the neuropathic pain severity is maximal when all nerve roots are avulsed [2, 17, 21, 55].

4. Medical treatment

This kind of pain, particularly in case of nerve root avulsions, is difficult to treat due to partial responses and frequent relapses [5, 6, 17]. The response to pharmacological treatments decreases when the pain intensity increases [6].

The non-steroidal anti-inflammatory drugs (NSAIDs) are of little help in the chronic phase [17, 30].

The first step is *tricyclic antidepressants (TCAs)* or *serotonin* and *noradrenaline reuptake inhibitors* [6, 57, 87]. Among TCAs, amitriptyline (25–125 mg/day) and venlafaxine (150–225 mg/day) are the most commonly used [6, 57]. They not only help with the pain but also with the accompanying nervous depression [57, 87]. A regular ECG surveillance is recommended as at high doses these drugs can induce cardiac arrhythmias [88]. Duloxetine, the most commonly used serotonin-noradrenaline reuptake inhibitor, is devoid of cholinergic or cardiac side effects [87].

The second step is the combination of the above-mentioned drugs with anti-epileptic agents [89], like *gabapentin* or *pregabalin* [6, 19, 27, 57, 87]. Clonazepam at night time is very effective, but it can induce drowsiness, and some patients find it difficult to tolerate [90]. Other anti-epileptic drugs like topiramate, carbamazepine, oxcarbazepine and lamotrigine are also used but with limited success [57].

Lidocaine (lignocaine) 5% patches applied to the painful area are the third line of medical treatment [27, 91, 92]. It controls the cold allodynia but not the mechanical one [73].

Capsaicin 8% patches are used but can cause severe local skin irritation [27].

Oral cannabinoids, which were successful in controlling brachial plexus injury pain in rats [70], have limited success in humans and are not currently recommended [93].

Opioids (tramadol [6, 89], morphine, oxycodone and tapentadol) are to be avoided as they are not very effective in the treatment of neuropathic pain [32] and because of their addictive properties [27, 57, 91, 92]. In any case the opioid dose should never exceed 180 mg/day of oral morphine equivalents [57] and should be complemented with TCAs and anti-epileptic drugs [89].

Other drugs have been tried experimentally in rats, like rapamycin [94], intrathecal Trichostatin A (TSA) [94] or intravenous immunoglobulin [95], but there are no reports of their use in humans.

Transcutaneous electrical nerve stimulation (TENS) has been used to control and prevent the development of neuropathic pain after brachial plexus injury [35, 96–98]. Its main advantage is that it can be self-applied by the patient. However, it needs constant application, and at times it can provoke local skin irritation [35, 96–98].

The common clinical features shared by neuropathic pain and CRPS hinder a pure clinical diagnosis [6]. Distinguishing between both of them is essential as the latter causes greater disabilities [99]. To differentiate them, an ultrasound examination can be performed, as the muscular architecture is preserved in neuropathic pain but not in CRPS [99].

Medical treatments can also classify the pain: *stellate ganglion blocks* will only relieve CRPS [6, 100, 101]. Other therapies for CRPS include *botulinum toxin,* which can be used to treat muscular trigger points [102] when found, and *electroacupuncture,* which has been found effective in controlling experimental brachial plexus pain in rats [103]. We have not found any publication reporting the use of electroacupuncture in human beings.

5. Surgical treatment

Brachial plexus injury repair by direct suture, by grafts or by nerve transfers, particularly sensory nerve transfers, minimizes the incidence and severity of neuropathic pain [4, 26, 34, 67, 104–109], and the sooner the repair is done the better [25, 67]. CRPS is the exception as further surgery outside trapped nerve decompression seems to have a negative impact on the outcome [101]. In these cases either an interscalene [102] or stellate ganglion block [110] or a cervical spinal cord stimulator [111–113] is recommended instead. The phantom limb pain only improves with central nervous system procedures [114, 115].

There are two main roads of action: neuromodulation and ablative procedures. The first group relies on applying electric impulses to different areas of the central or peripheral nervous system, aiming to block the transmission of the nerve impulses that are finally interpreted as pain in the sensory motor cortex. They are particularly effective for continuous pain but less so for paroxysmal painful discharges [84]. The ablative procedures aim to destroy the posterior horn spinal cord neurons that start to fire in an abnormal way after being disconnected from their peripheral sensory input [25, 64–66], controlling paroxysmal pain better than continuous pain [84].

5.1. Neuromodulation procedures

Peripheral nerve stimulation provides 50–83% pain relief in 65–80% of the patients [116–120], and the affected limb preserves the residual function remaining after the injury [121]. Allodynia and neuropathic pain are controlled with mild improvement in the sensory function [116, 118]. The results are stable long-term [118, 119, 121]. The electrodes can be implanted with an open surgical procedure [117, 119] or percutaneously under ultrasound guidance [116, 120]. Unfortunately lead fracture, displacement or infection can spoil an initial successful result [116, 120]. A further refinement is to apply the stimulating electrodes not through a cuff around the affected nerve but by direct selective nerve fascicle stimulation [122]. In this way only the affected sensory fascicles are stimulated and not the motor ones, improving the results and reducing the side effects, particularly muscle spasms [122].

Cervical spinal cord stimulation stops the transmission of the abnormal electrical impulses coming from the deafferented posterior spinal cord horn neurons [123], controlling the pain with preservation of the remaining upper limb function [112, 124, 125]. Its success rate in the treatment of neuropathic pain associated with brachial plexus injuries is 50% [51, 111–113, 124–129]. It is particularly useful in CRPS [112] but it also helpful in nerve root avulsions [129]. In cases of failed previous dorsal root entry zone (DREZ), lesioning can provide good pain control [113]. Contrariwise, when the spinal cord stimulation failed the DREZ-otomy through radiofrequency, it yields suboptimal results [130]. Nevertheless several research groups recommend to restrict the cervical spinal cord stimulation for failed previous DREZ-otomy due to its high economical costs [25, 131–133]. A trial period is needed before the definitive pulse generator implantation to predict the results [129]. The stimulation parameters can be modified according to the patient's individual needs through an external programming device. The electrodes can be implanted percutaneously or surgically. Lead fracture or dislocation and battery exhaustion will require surgical revision of the system. Some patients experience discomfort due to paresthesias particularly when rotating the head [111, 124]. This can be minimized by reprograming the active electrodes and the intensity of the electrical stimuli.

Pulsed radiofrequency has been reported in a few cases of brachial plexus injury including one with concomitant limb amputation, with a 60–70% pain improvement in a 6-month follow-up [38, 134]. The main advantage is that radiofrequency does not induce additional motor or sensory deficit, although the results are not long-lasting [135]. The data are insufficient to draw any definitive conclusions [38, 134, 135].

In small clinical series of patients, *deep brain stimulation* has shown a 55% improvement in neuropathic pain arising from brachial plexus injury and traumatic amputation pain [20, 58, 136]. After 1 year the effectivity is reduced in many patients, and increasing the intensity of the electrical stimuli is not always successful to improve the deteriorating results [20]. There is no agreement on where is the best target for the stimulation: some recommend the sensory thalamus [20, 58] and others the periaqueductal grey matter [137, 138].

In neuropathic pain induced by brachial plexus injury, *motor cortex stimulation* has shown a 42% effectiveness in controlling the continuous pain but no effectiveness for the paroxysmal discharges [84, 139]. A major drawback is the lack of factors to be able to predict the results to be expected [84]. This is particularly important considering the high cost and surgical risks involved in this technology.

5.2. Ablative procedures

The medial thalamotomy, the spinothalamic tractotomy, and the anterolateral tractotomy have been abandoned due to the limited pain control they provide and the side effects they carry [119].

The DREZ is an anatomical area of the spinal cord composed by the dorsal rootlets, Lissauer's tract and the dorsal horn [25]. *DREZ-otomy* aims to destroy the neurons located in the posterior horn of the spinal cord that start firing abnormally once deprived of their peripheral sensory input [25, 140]. It has proved particularly effective in the control of brachial plexus-induced neuropathic pain [22, 23, 28, 48, 140, 141], but it is a destructive procedure that can be applied when no residual upper limb function has to be preserved (i.e. nerve root avulsions). It is particularly effective in controlling the paroxysmal pain but not so much in the constant aspect of it [23–25, 84, 133, 139, 142]. It provides a better pain control than the neuromodulation procedures, with a reported long-term success rates of 50–75% [22, 25, 29, 48, 143]. Unfortunately about 10% of patients develop ipsilateral leg weakness and ataxia [22–24, 28, 48, 133, 140, 141] due to the vicinity of the area to be lesioned to the motor corticospinal tract laterally and the dorsal column with proprioceptive information medially [25, 140]. This successful pain control correlates with an improvement in anxiety and depression and in a third of patients in returning to work [133, 144]. The pain improvement with this technique is independent of the time elapsed since the injury and the DREZ-otomy [25, 133]. Pain recurrence is expected in 13–20% of the patients [22, 23, 25, 28, 29, 132, 143, 145–147] particularly in those with constant type of pain [23, 24, 139] but with an acceptable pain control in over 60% of them [132, 143].

The recurrences seem to be more common in the first 12 months post-op and much rarer after 5 years of follow-up [48, 132]. Pain control and recurrences seem to be less common among nerve root avulsions than with other more peripheral brachial plexus injuries [143, 145]. Some surgeons have considered that a bad result would mean a DREZ lesion of insufficient size [25, 131] and used the intraoperative ultrasound imaging to guide the shape and size of those lesions [131]. They reported an initial 100% pain control that decreased to 87% on 47.5 months follow-up but at the price of a higher rate of lower extremity weakness and ataxia [131] (17%, compared to 10% in other patient series [22–24, 28, 48, 140, 141]). These results also reflect that apart from the spinal cord, there are other higher central nervous system areas involved in the generation and maintenance of the neuropathic pain induced after brachial plexus injury [148].

Lack of DREZ region damage confirmed in preoperative MRI seems to be an indicator of successful pain control with the DREZ procedure to the point that no patient with spinal cord dorsal horn abnormalities had a completely pain-free outcome [22]. It is suggested that if the posterior horn is abnormal, the thalamus will most likely develop deafferented neurons that will start firing in an abnormal pattern and thus the treatment should be directed there and not to the spinal cord [22]. This observation contradicts the fact that surgically amputated patients due to different medical conditions in whom a normal spinal cord anatomy is preserved fare worse with the DREZ operation than those that had a traumatic amputation [115]. In these DREZ-otomy failed cases, a cervical spinal cord stimulator is recommended [113]. Post-operative MRI examinations in radiofrequency DREZ lesions have shown that the surgically lesioned area extends beyond the posterior horn [149]. This is in concordance with the clinical fact that some patients develop post-operative leg weakness, ataxia and sensory abnormalities below the operated area [22–24, 28, 48, 133, 140, 141].

DREZ-otomy provides 83% pain control rate in phantom pain [115, 150, 151], 67% in burning pain and 29% for stump pain [115, 152]. Both amputation and nerve root avulsion phantom pain seem to benefit from DREZ-otomies [115, 150, 151]. The results in pain improvement are better in traumatic amputations than in those due to medical conditions [28, 115]. Some researchers recommend to start with neurostimulation in phantom limb pain and to recourse to the DREZ-otomy as a last resort [152].

The DREZ-otomy can be created microsurgicaly (Sindou's technique) [25], with radiofrequency (Nashold's technique) [29, 48], with laser [153–156] or even with an ultrasonic microprobe [131], but there are no major differences in pain control or patients' quality of life between them [142, 156]. The microsurgical technique is performed with the regular bipolar forceps, which is less expensive than the other options (radiofrequency, laser, ultrasonic probe), making it ideal for countries with limited resources [144, 157]. Some scientists have attempted intraoperative neurophysiological monitoring to improve the clinical results [65, 158, 159]. Freeing the spinal cord completely helps to stop pain induction with neck movements [25]. A concern that has not yet been studied in detail is the possible long-term effects of extensive cervical laminectomies required for the procedure, as it might accelerate cervical kyphotic deformity with cervical spinal cord myelopathy [147]. In any case the original full bilateral cervical C_5-T_1 laminectomies [25, 140] have been replaced in many surgical units by hemi-laminectomies.

6. Conclusions

Brachial plexus injuries can be the source of chronic pain. This pain can be neuropathic, CRPS and/or phantom limb, particularly if there is extensive nerve root avulsion or an upper limb amputation. The pain is oftentimes excruciating and leads to a bad quality of life even interfering with the physiotherapy needed to achieve a good recovery. The response to treatment of this pain is not always as successful as expected. Some patients respond to medication, but many need neuromodulation or ablative procedures. The most effective surgical technique is the DREZ-otomy, but 10% of patients develop side effects. If the ablative procedures fail, cervical spinal cord stimulation can be attempted.

Author details

Nieves Saiz-Sapena[1*], Vicente Vanaclocha-Vanaclocha[2], José María Ortiz-Criado[3], L. Vanaclocha[4] and Nieves Vanaclocha[5]

*Address all correspondence to: nssapena@hotmail.com

1 Hospital 9 de Octubre, Valencia, Spain

2 Department of Neurosurgery, Hospital General Universitario, Valencia, Spain

3 Universidad Católica San Vicente Mártir, Valencia, Spain

4 iBSc in Clinical Sciences, UCL School of Medicine, London, United Kingdom

5 Medical School, University College London, London, United Kingdom

References

[1] Sinha S, Pemmaiah D, Midha R. Management of brachial plexus injuries in adults: Clinical evaluation and diagnosis. Neurology India. 2015;**63**(6):918-925

[2] Tantigate D, Wongtrakul S, Vathana T, Limthongthang R, Songcharoen P. Neuropathic pain in brachial plexus injury. Hand Surgery: An International Journal Devoted to Hand and Upper Limb Surgery and Related Research: Journal of the Asia-Pacific Federation of Societies for Hand Therapy. 2015;**20**(1):39-45. DOI: 10.1142/S0218810415500057

[3] Ciaramitaro P, Padua L, Devigili G, et al. Prevalence of neuropathic pain in patients with traumatic brachial plexus injury: A multicenter prospective hospital-based study. Pain Medicine (Malden, Mass.). 2017;**18**(12):2428-2432. DOI: 10.1093/pm/pnw360

[4] Berman JS, Birch R, Anand P. Pain following human brachial plexus injury with spinal cord root avulsion and the effect of surgery. Pain. 1998;**75**(2-3):199-207

[5] Santana MVB, Bina MT, Paz MG, et al. High prevalence of neuropathic pain in the hand of patients with traumatic brachial plexus injury: A cross-sectional study. Arquivos de Neuro-Psiquiatria. 2016;**74**(11):895-901. DOI: 10.1590/0004-282X20160149

[6] Subedi A, Chaudakshetrin P, Chotisukarat H, Mandee S. Effect of co-morbid conditions on persistent neuropathic pain after brachial plexus injury in adult patients. Journal of Clinical Neurology (Seoul, Korea). 2016;**12**(4):489-494. DOI: 10.3988/jcn.2016.12.4.489

[7] Teixeira MJ, da Paz MG da S, Bina MT, et al. Neuropathic pain after brachial plexus avulsion—Central and peripheral mechanisms. BMC Neurology. 2015;**15**:73. DOI: 10.1186/s12883-015-0329-x

[8] Dengler NF, Antoniadis G, Grolik B, Wirtz CR, König R, Pedro MT. Mechanisms, treatment, and patient outcome of iatrogenic injury to the brachial plexus—A retrospective single-center study. World Neurosurgery. 2017;**107**:868-876. DOI: 10.1016/j.wneu.2017.08.119

[9] Carofino BC, Brogan DM, Kircher MF, et al. Iatrogenic nerve injuries during shoulder surgery. The Journal of Bone and Joint Surgery. American Volume. 2013;**95**(18):1667-1674. DOI: 10.2106/JBJS.L.00238

[10] Desai KR, Nemcek AA. Iatrogenic brachial plexopathy due to improper positioning during radiofrequency ablation. Seminars in Interventional Radiology. 2011;**28**(2):167-170. DOI: 10.1055/s-0031-1280657

[11] Guedes-Corrêa JF, Pereira MR da C, Torrão-Junior FJL, Martins JV, Barbosa DAN. A neglected cause of iatrogenic brachial plexus injuries in psychiatric patients. Neurosurgery. 1 Mar 2018;**82**(3):307-311. DOI: 10.1093/neuros/nyx162

[12] Joiner ERA, Skaggs DL, Arkader A, et al. Iatrogenic nerve injuries in the treatment of supracondylar humerus fractures: Are we really just missing nerve injuries on preoperative examination? Journal of Pediatric Orthopedics. 2014;**34**(4):388-392. DOI: 10.1097/BPO.0000000000000171

[13] Po BT, Hansen HR. Iatrogenic brachial plexus injury: survey of the literature and of pertinent cases. Anesthesia and Analgesia. 1969;**48**(6):915-922

[14] Scully WF, Wilson DJ, Parada SA, Arrington ED. Iatrogenic nerve injuries in shoulder surgery. The Journal of the American Academy of Orthopaedic Surgeons. 2013;**21**(12): 717-726. DOI: 10.5435/JAAOS-21-12-717

[15] Rasulić L, Savić A, Vitošević F, et al. Iatrogenic peripheral nerve injuries-surgical treatment and outcome: 10 Years' experience. World Neurosurgery. 2017;**103**:841-851.e6. DOI: 10.1016/j.wneu.2017.04.099

[16] Antoniadis G, Kretschmer T, Pedro MT, König RW, Heinen CPG, Richter H-P. Iatrogenic nerve injuries: Prevalence, diagnosis and treatment. Deutsches Ärzteblatt International. 2014;**111**(16):273-279. DOI: 10.3238/arztebl.2014.0273

[17] Zhou Y, Liu P, Rui J, Zhao X, Lao J. The clinical characteristics of neuropathic pain in patients with total brachial plexus avulsion: A 30-case study. Injury. 2016;**47**(8): 1719-1724. DOI: 10.1016/j.injury.2016.05.022

[18] Park SH, Esquenazi Y, Kline DG, Kim DH. Surgical outcomes of 156 spinal accessory nerve injuries caused by lymph node biopsy procedures. Journal of Neurosurgery: Spine. 2015;**23**(4):518-525. DOI: 10.3171/2014.12.SPINE14968

[19] Shibahara H, Okubo K, Takeshita N, Nishimura D. Medical treatment including pregabalin and radiation therapy provided remarkable relief for neuropathic pain by brachial plexus invasion in a patient with esophageal cancer. Gan to Kagaku Ryoho. 2012;**39**(2): 277-280

[20] Abreu V, Vaz R, Rebelo V, et al. Thalamic deep brain stimulation for neuropathic pain: Efficacy at three years' follow-up. Neuromodulation: Journal of the International Neuromodulation Society. 2017;**20**(5):504-513. DOI: 10.1111/ner.12620

[21] Bertelli JA, Ghizoni MF, Loure Iro Chaves DP. Sensory disturbances and pain complaints after brachial plexus root injury: A prospective study involving 150 adult patients. Microsurgery. 2011;**31**(2):93-97. DOI: 10.1002/micr.20832

[22] Ko AL, Ozpinar A, Raskin JS, Magill ST, Raslan AM, Burchiel KJ. Correlation of preoperative MRI with the long-term outcomes of dorsal root entry zone lesioning for brachial plexus avulsion pain. Journal of Neurosurgery. 2016;**124**(5):1470-1478. DOI: 10.3171/2015.2.JNS142572

[23] Aichaoui F, Mertens P, Sindou M. Dorsal root entry zone lesioning for pain after brachial plexus avulsion: Results with special emphasis on differential effects on the paroxysmal versus the continuous components. A prospective study in a 29-patient consecutive series. Pain. 2011;**152**(8):1923-1930. DOI: 10.1016/j.pain.2011.03.037

[24] Haninec P, Sámal F, Tomás R, Houstava L, Dubovwý P. Direct repair (nerve grafting), neurotization, and end-to-side neurorrhaphy in the treatment of brachial plexus injury. Journal of Neurosurgery. 2007;**106**(3):391-399. DOI: 10.3171/jns.2007.106.3.391

[25] Sindou MP, Blondet E, Emery E, Mertens P. Microsurgical lesioning in the dorsal root entry zone for pain due to brachial plexus avulsion: A prospective series of 55 patients. Journal of Neurosurgery. 2005;**102**(6):1018-1028. DOI: 10.3171/jns.2005.102.6.1018

[26] Htut M, Misra P, Anand P, Birch R, Carlstedt T. Pain phenomena and sensory recovery following brachial plexus avulsion injury and surgical repairs. Journal of Hand Surgery (Edinburgh, Scotland). 2006;**31**(6):596-605. DOI: 10.1016/j.jhsb.2006.04.027

[27] Finnerup NB, Norrbrink C, Fuglsang-Frederiksen A, Terkelsen AJ, Hojlund AP, Jensen TS. Pain, referred sensations, and involuntary muscle movements in brachial plexus injury. Acta Neurologica Scandinavica. 2010;**121**(5):320-327. DOI: 10.1111/j.1600-0404.2009.01248.x

[28] Awad AJ, Forbes JA, Jermakowicz W, Eli IM, Blumenkopf B, Konrad P. Experience with 25 years of dorsal root entry zone lesioning at a single institution. Surgical Neurology International. 2013;**4**:64. DOI: 10.4103/2152-7806.112182

[29] Friedman AH, Nashold BS, Bronec PR. Dorsal root entry zone lesions for the treatment of brachial plexus avulsion injuries: A follow-up study. Neurosurgery. 1988;**22**(2):369-373

[30] Zhou Y, Liu P, Rui J, Zhao X, Lao J. The associated factors and clinical features of neuropathic pain after brachial plexus injuries: A cross-sectional study. The Clinical Journal of Pain. 2017;**33**(11):1030-1036. DOI: 10.1097/AJP.0000000000000493

[31] Privat JM, Allieu Y, Bonnel F, De Godebout J. Pain following traumatic lesions of the brachial plexus (radicular avulsions and truncular lesions). Neuro-Chirurgie. 1985;**31**(5): 435-441

[32] Bruxelle J, Travers V, Thiebaut JB. Occurrence and treatment of pain after brachial plexus injury. Clinical Orthopaedics. 1988;(237):87-95

[33] Woolf CJ. Dissecting out mechanisms responsible for peripheral neuropathic pain: Implications for diagnosis and therapy. Life Sciences. 2004;**74**(21):2605-2610. DOI: 10.1016/j.lfs.2004.01.003

[34] Bonilla G, Di Masi G, Battaglia D, Otero JM, Socolovsky M. Pain and brachial plexus lesions: Evaluation of initial outcomes after reconstructive microsurgery and validation of a new pain severity scale. Acta Neurochirurgica. 2011;**153**(1):171-176. DOI: 10.1007/s00701-010-0709-3

[35] Parry CB. Pain in avulsion of the brachial plexus. Neurosurgery. 1984;**15**(6):960-965

[36] Zorub DS, Nashold BS, Cook WA. Avulsion of the brachial plexus. I. A review with implications on the therapy of intractable pain. Surgical Neurology. 1974;**2**(5):347-353

[37] Malin JP, Winkelmüller W. Phantom phenomena (phantom arm) following cervical root avulsion. Effect of dorsal root entry zone thermocoagulation. European Archives of Psychiatry and Neurological Sciences. 1985;**235**(1):53-56

[38] Zheng B, Song L, Liu H. Pulsed radiofrequency of brachial plexus under ultrasound guidance for refractory stump pain: A case report. Journal of Pain Research. 2017;**10**:2601-2604. DOI: 10.2147/JPR.S148479

[39] Al-Qattan MM. Self-mutilation in children with obstetric brachial plexus palsy. Journal of Hand Surgery (Edinburgh, Scotland). 1999;**24**(5):547-549. DOI: 10.1054/jhsb.1999.0222

[40] McCann ME, Waters P, Goumnerova LC, Berde C. Self-mutilation in young children following brachial plexus birth injury. Pain. 2004;**110**(1-2):123-129. DOI: 10.1016/j.pain.2004.03.020

[41] Oskay D, Oksüz C, Akel S, Firat T, Leblebicioğlu G. Quality of life in mothers of children with obstetrical brachial plexus palsy. Pediatrics International : Official Journal of the Japan Pediatric Society. 2012;**54**(1):117-122. DOI: 10.1111/j.1442-200X.2011.03455.x

[42] Rasulić L, Savić A, Živković B, et al. Outcome after brachial plexus injury surgery and impact on quality of life. Acta Neurochirurgica. 2017;**159**(7):1257-1264. DOI: 10.1007/s00701-017-3205-1

[43] Bailey R, Kaskutas V, Fox I, Baum CM, Mackinnon SE. Effect of upper extremity nerve damage on activity participation, pain, depression, and quality of life. Journal of Hand Surgery. 2009;**34**(9):1682-1688. DOI: 10.1016/j.jhsa.2009.07.002

[44] Choi PD, Novak CB, Mackinnon SE, Kline DG. Quality of life and functional outcome following brachial plexus injury. Journal of Hand Surgery. 1997;**22**(4):605-612. DOI: 10.1016/S0363-5023(97)80116-5

[45] Terzis JK, Kostopoulos VK. The surgical treatment of brachial plexus injuries in adults. Plastic and Reconstructive Surgery. 2007;**119**(4):73e-92e. DOI: 10.1097/01.prs.0000254859.51903.97

[46] Raducha JE, Cohen B, Blood T, Katarincic JA. Review of brachial plexus birth palsy: Injury and rehabilitation. Rhode Island Medical Journal (2013). 2017;**100**(11):17-21

[47] Carvalho GA, Nikkhah G, Matthies C, Penkert G, Samii M. Diagnosis of root avulsions in traumatic brachial plexus injuries: Value of computerized tomography myelography and magnetic resonance imaging. Journal of Neurosurgery. 1997;**86**(1):69-76. DOI: 10.3171/jns.1997.86.1.0069

[48] Rawlings CE, el-Naggar AO, Nashold BS. The DREZ procedure: An update on technique. British Journal of Neurosurgery. 1989;**3**(6):633-642

[49] Vannier J-L, Belkheyar Z, Oberlin C, Montravers P. Management of neuropathic pain after brachial plexus injury in adult patients: A report of 60 cases. Annales Françaises d'Anesthèsie et de Rèanimation. 2008;**27**(11):890-895. DOI: 10.1016/j.annfar.2008.08.013

[50] Giuffre JL, Bishop AT, Spinner RJ, Shin AY. Surgical technique of a partial tibial nerve transfer to the tibialis anterior motor branch for the treatment of peroneal nerve injury. Annals of Plastic Surgery. 2012;**69**(1):48-53. DOI: 10.1097/SAP.0b013e31824c94e5

[51] Brill S, Aryeh IG. Neuromodulation in the management of pain from brachial plexus injury. Pain Physician. 2008;**11**(1):81-85

[52] Le Feuvre P, Aldington D. Know pain know gain: proposing a treatment approach for phantom limb pain. Journal of the Royal Army Medical Corps. 2014;**160**(1):16-21. DOI: 10.1136/jramc-2013-000141

[53] Hall GC, Carroll D, Parry D, McQuay HJ. Epidemiology and treatment of neuropathic pain: The UK primary care perspective. Pain. 2006;**122**(1-2):156-162. DOI: 10.1016/j.pain.2006.01.030

[54] Jensen TS, Krebs B, Nielsen J, Rasmussen P. Immediate and long-term phantom limb pain in amputees: Incidence, clinical characteristics and relationship to pre-amputation limb pain. Pain. 1985;**21**(3):267-278

[55] Shankar H, Hansen J, Thomas K. Phantom pain in a patient with brachial plexus avulsion injury. Pain Medicine (Malden, Mass.). 2015;**16**(4):777-781. DOI: 10.1111/pme.12635

[56] Jensen TS, Baron R, Haanpää M, et al. A new definition of neuropathic pain. Pain. 2011;**152**(10):2204-2205. DOI: 10.1016/j.pain.2011.06.017

[57] Murnion BP. Neuropathic pain: Current definition and review of drug treatment. Australian Prescriber. 2018;**41**(3):60-63. DOI: 10.18773/austprescr.2018.022

[58] Pereira EAC, Boccard SG, Linhares P, et al. Thalamic deep brain stimulation for neuropathic pain after amputation or brachial plexus avulsion. Neurosurgical Focus. 2013; **35**(3):E7. DOI: 10.3171/2013.7.FOCUS1346

[59] Schwartzman RJ, Grothusen JR. Brachial plexus traction injury: Quantification of sensory abnormalities. Pain Medicine (Malden, Mass.). 2008;**9**(7):950-957. DOI: 10.1111/j.1526-4637.2007.00394.x

[60] Guenot M, Hupe JM, Mertens P, Ainsworth A, Bullier J, Sindou M. A new type of microelectrode for obtaining unitary recordings in the human spinal cord. Journal of Neurosurgery. 1999;**91**(1 Suppl):25-32

[61] Loeser JD, Ward AA, White LE. Chronic deafferentation of human spinal cord neurons. Journal of Neurosurgery. 1968;**29**(1):48-50. DOI: 10.3171/jns.1968.29.1.0048

[62] Fujioka H, Shimoji K, Tomita M, Denda S, Hokari T, Tohyama M. Effects of dorsal root entry zone lesion on spinal cord potentials evoked by segmental, ascending and descending volleys. Acta Neurochirurgica. 1992;**117**(3-4):135-142

[63] Guenot M, Bullier J, Sindou M. Clinical and electrophysiological expression of deafferentation pain alleviated by dorsal root entry zone lesions in rats. Journal of Neurosurgery. 2002;**97**(6):1402-1409. DOI: 10.3171/jns.2002.97.6.1402

[64] Jeanmonod D, Sindou M, Mauguière F. Intraoperative electrophysiological recordings during microsurgical DREZ-tomies in man. Stereotactic and Functional Neurosurgery 1990;54-55:80-85. doi:10.1159/000100195

[65] Falci S, Best L, Bayles R, Lammertse D, Starnes C. Dorsal root entry zone microcoagulation for spinal cord injury-related central pain: Operative intramedullary electrophysiological guidance and clinical outcome. Journal of Neurosurgery. 2002;**97**(2 Suppl):193-200

[66] Loeser JD, Ward AA. Some effects of deafferentation on neurons of the cat spinal cord. Archives of Neurology. 1967;**17**(6):629-636

[67] Bertelli JA, Ghizoni MF. Pain after avulsion injuries and complete palsy of the brachial plexus: The possible role of nonavulsed roots in pain generation. Neurosurgery. 2008;**62**(5):1104-1114. DOI: 10.1227/01.neu.0000325872.37258.12

[68] Mika J, Zychowska M, Popiolek-Barczyk K, Rojewska E, Przewlocka B. Importance of glial activation in neuropathic pain. European Journal of Pharmacology. 2013;**716**(1-3):106-119. DOI: 10.1016/j.ejphar.2013.01.072

[69] Liu Y, Wang L, Meng C, Zhou Y, Lao J, Zhao X. A new model for the study of neuropathic pain after brachial plexus injury. Injury. 2017;**48**(2):253-261. DOI: 10.1016/j.injury.2016.11.007

[70] Paszcuk AF, Dutra RC, da Silva KABS, Quintão NLM, Campos MM, Calixto JB. Cannabinoid agonists inhibit neuropathic pain induced by brachial plexus avulsion in mice by affecting glial cells and MAP kinases. PLoS One. 2011;**6**(9):e24034. DOI: 10.1371/journal.pone.0024034

[71] Iwasaki R, Matsuura Y, Ohtori S, Suzuki T, Kuniyoshi K, Takahashi K. Activation of astrocytes and microglia in the C3-T4 dorsal horn by lower trunk avulsion in a rat

model of neuropathic pain. Journal of Hand Surgery. 2013;**38**(5):841-846. DOI: 10.1016/j.jhsa.2013.01.034

[72] Clark AK, Old EA, Malcangio M. Neuropathic pain and cytokines: Current perspectives. Journal of Pain Research. 2013;**6**:803-814. DOI: 10.2147/JPR.S53660

[73] Rodrigues-Filho R, Santos ARS, Bertelli JA, Calixto JB. Avulsion injury of the rat brachial plexus triggers hyperalgesia and allodynia in the hindpaws: A new model for the study of neuropathic pain. Brain Research. 2003;**982**(2):186-194

[74] Rinaldi PC, Young RF, Albe-Fessard D, Chodakiewitz J. Spontaneous neuronal hyperactivity in the medial and intralaminar thalamic nuclei of patients with deafferentation pain. Journal of Neurosurgery. 1991;**74**(3):415-421. DOI: 10.3171/jns.1991.74.3.0415

[75] Grüsser SM, Mühlnickel W, Schaefer M, et al. Remote activation of referred phantom sensation and cortical reorganization in human upper extremity amputees. Experimental Brain Research. 2004;**154**(1):97-102. DOI: 10.1007/s00221-003-1649-4

[76] Tasker RR, Gorecki J, Lenz FA, Hirayama T, Dostrovsky JO. Thalamic microelectrode recording and microstimulation in central and deafferentation pain. Applied Neurophysiology. 1987;**50**(1-6):414-417

[77] Jeanmonod D, Magnin M, Morel A. Thalamus and neurogenic pain: Physiological, anatomical and clinical data. Neuroreport. 1993;**4**(5):475-478

[78] Zhang L, Zhang Y, Zhao Z-Q. Anterior cingulate cortex contributes to the descending facilitatory modulation of pain via dorsal reticular nucleus. The European Journal of Neuroscience. 2005;**22**(5):1141-1148. DOI: 10.1111/j.1460-9568.2005.04302.x

[79] Kim CH, Oh Y, Chung JM, Chung K. The changes in expression of three subtypes of TTX sensitive sodium channels in sensory neurons after spinal nerve ligation. Brain Research. Molecular Brain Research. 2001;**95**(1-2):153-161

[80] Campbell JN, Meyer RA. Mechanisms of neuropathic pain. Neuron. 2006;**52**(1):77-92. DOI: 10.1016/j.neuron.2006.09.021

[81] Nickel FT, Seifert F, Lanz S, Maihöfner C. Mechanisms of neuropathic pain. European Neuropsychopharmacology: Journal of the European College of Neuropsychopharmacology. 2012;**22**(2):81-91. DOI: 10.1016/j.euroneuro.2011.05.005

[82] Woolf CJ, Shortland P, Coggeshall RE. Peripheral nerve injury triggers central sprouting of myelinated afferents. Nature. 1992;**355**(6355):75-78. DOI: 10.1038/355075a0

[83] Guenot M, Bullier J, Rospars J-P, Lansky P, Mertens P, Sindou M. Single-unit analysis of the spinal dorsal horn in patients with neuropathic pain. Journal of Clinical Neurophysiology. 2003;**20**(2):143-150

[84] Ali M, Saitoh Y, Oshino S, et al. Differential efficacy of electric motor cortex stimulation and lesioning of the dorsal root entry zone for continuous vs paroxysmal pain after brachial plexus avulsion. Neurosurgery. 2011;**68**(5):1252-1258. DOI: 10.1227/NEU.0b013e31820c04a9

[85] Makin TR, Scholz J, Filippini N, Henderson Slater D, Tracey I, Johansen-Berg H. Phantom pain is associated with preserved structure and function in the former hand area. Nature Communications. 2013;**4**:1570. DOI: 10.1038/ncomms2571

[86] Karl A, Birbaumer N, Lutzenberger W, Cohen LG, Flor H. Reorganization of motor and somatosensory cortex in upper extremity amputees with phantom limb pain. Journal of Neuroscience: The Official Journal of the Society for Neuroscience. 2001;**21**(10):3609-3618

[87] Finnerup NB, Attal N, Haroutounian S, et al. Pharmacotherapy for neuropathic pain in adults: A systematic review and meta-analysis. Lancet Neurology. 2015;**14**(2):162-173. DOI: 10.1016/S1474-4422(14)70251-0

[88] Davis G, Curtin CM. Management of pain in complex nerve injuries. Hand Clinics. 2016;**32**(2):257-262. DOI: 10.1016/j.hcl.2015.12.011

[89] Moulin D, Boulanger A, Clark AJ, et al. Pharmacological management of chronic neuropathic pain: Revised consensus statement from the Canadian Pain Society. Pain Research & Management. 2014;**19**(6):328-335

[90] Corrigan R, Derry S, Wiffen PJ, Moore RA. Clonazepam for neuropathic pain and fibromyalgia in adults. Cochrane Database of Systematic Reviews. 2012;**5**:CD009486. DOI: 10.1002/14651858.CD009486.pub2

[91] Provinciali L, Lattanzi S, Chiarlone R, et al. Topical pharmacologic approach with 5% lidocaine medicated plaster in the treatment of localized neuropathic pain. Minerva Medica. 2014;**105**(6):515-527

[92] Krumova EK, Zeller M, Westermann A, Maier C. Lidocaine patch (5%) produces a selective, but incomplete block of Aδ and C fibers. Pain. 2012;**153**(2):273-280. DOI: 10.1016/j.pain.2011.08.020

[93] Boychuk DG, Goddard G, Mauro G, Orellana MF. The effectiveness of cannabinoids in the management of chronic nonmalignant neuropathic pain: A systematic review. Journal of Oral & Facial Pain and Headache. 2015;**29**(1):7-14

[94] Zhao Y, Wu T. Histone deacetylase inhibition inhibits brachial plexus avulsion-induced neuropathic pain. Muscle & Nerve. 2018;**58**(3):434-440. DOI: 10.1002/mus.26160

[95] Morishima R, Nagaoka U, Nagao M, Isozaki E. Chronic brachial plexus neuritis that developed into typical neuralgic amyotrophy and positively responded to immunotherapy. Internal Medicine (Tokyo, Japan). 2018;**57**(7):1021-1026. DOI: 10.2169/internalmedicine.9482-17

[96] Goroszeniuk T, Pang D. Peripheral neuromodulation: A review. Current Pain and Headache Reports. 2014;**18**(5):412. DOI: 10.1007/s11916-014-0412-9

[97] Chakravarthy K, Nava A, Christo PJ, Williams K. Review of recent advances in peripheral nerve stimulation (PNS). Current Pain and Headache Reports. 2016;**20**(11):60. DOI: 10.1007/s11916-016-0590-8

[98] DeSantana JM, Walsh DM, Vance C, Rakel BA, Sluka KA. Effectiveness of transcutaneous electrical nerve stimulation for treatment of hyperalgesia and pain. Current Rheumatology Reports. 2008;**10**(6):492-499

[99] Vas L, Pai R. Musculoskeletal ultrasonography to distinguish muscle changes in complex regional pain syndrome type 1 from those of neuropathic pain: An observational study. Pain Practice: The Official Journal of World Institute of Pain. 2016;**16**(1):E1-E13. DOI: 10.1111/papr.12338

[100] Zinboonyahgoon N, Vlassakov K, Abrecht CR, Srinivasan S, Narang S. Brachial plexus block for cancer-related pain: A case series. Pain Physician. 2015;**18**(5):E917-E924

[101] Toshniwal G, Sunder R, Thomas R, Dureja GP. Management of complex regional pain syndrome type I in upper extremity-evaluation of continuous stellate ganglion block and continuous infraclavicular brachial plexus block: A pilot study. Pain Medicine (Malden, Mass.). 2012;**13**(1):96-106. DOI: 10.1111/j.1526-4637.2011.01285.x

[102] Fallatah SMA. Successful management of complex regional pain syndrome type 1 using single injection interscalene brachial plexus block. Saudi Journal of Anaesthesia. 2014;**8**(4):559-561. DOI: 10.4103/1658-354X.140903

[103] Liu H, Qian X-Y, An J-X, et al. Analgesic effects and neuropathology changes of electroacupuncture on curing a rat model of brachial plexus neuralgia induced by cobra venom. Pain Physician. 2016;**19**(3):E435-E447

[104] Bertelli JA. Distal sensory nerve transfers in lower-type injuries of the brachial plexus. Journal of Hand Surgery. 2012;**37**(6):1194-1199. DOI: 10.1016/j.jhsa.2012.02.047

[105] Kato N, Htut M, Taggart M, Carlstedt T, Birch R. The effects of operative delay on the relief of neuropathic pain after injury to the brachial plexus: A review of 148 cases. Journal of Bone and Joint Surgery. British Volume (London). 2006;**88**(6):756-759. DOI: 10.1302/0301-620X.88B6.16995

[106] Anand P, Birch R. Restoration of sensory function and lack of long-term chronic pain syndromes after brachial plexus injury in human neonates. Brain: A Journal of Neurology. 2002;**125**(Pt 1):113-122

[107] Ho ES, Curtis CG, Clarke HM. Pain in children following microsurgical reconstruction for obstetrical brachial plexus palsy. Journal of Hand Surgery. 2015;**40**(6):1177-1183. DOI: 10.1016/j.jhsa.2015.02.003

[108] Mohammad-Reda A. Early post-operative results after repair of traumatic brachial plexus palsy. Turkish Neurosurgery. 2013;**23**(1):1-9. DOI: 10.5137/1019-5149.JTN.5654-11.3

[109] Berman J, Anand P, Chen L, Taggart M, Birch R. Pain relief from preganglionic injury to the brachial plexus by late intercostal nerve transfer. Journal of Bone and Joint Surgery. British Volume (London). 1996;**78**(5):759-760

[110] Datta R, Agrawal J, Sharma A, Rathore VS, Datta S. A study of the efficacy of stellate ganglion blocks in complex regional pain syndromes of the upper body. Journal

of Anaesthesiology Clinical Pharmacology. 2017;**33**(4):534-540. DOI: 10.4103/joacp.JOACP_326_16

[111] Deer TR, Skaribas IM, Haider N, et al. Effectiveness of cervical spinal cord stimulation for the management of chronic pain. Neuromodulation: Journal of the International Neuromodulation Society. 2014;**17**(3):265-271; discussion 271. DOI: 10.1111/ner.12119

[112] Chang Chien GC, Candido KD, Saeed K, Knezevic NN. Cervical spinal cord stimulation treatment of deafferentation pain from brachial plexus avulsion injury complicated by complex regional pain syndrome. Case Reports. 2014;**3**(3):29-34. DOI: 10.1213/XAA.0000000000000041

[113] Lai H-Y, Lee C-Y, Lee S-T. High cervical spinal cord stimulation after failed dorsal root entry zone surgery for brachial plexus avulsion pain. Surgical Neurology. 2009;**72**(3):286-289; discussion 289. DOI: 10.1016/j.surneu.2008.06.019

[114] Parmar VK, Gee L, Smith H, Pilitsis JG. Supraspinal stimulation for treatment of refractory pain. Clinical Neurology and Neurosurgery. 2014;**123**:155-163. DOI: 10.1016/j.clineuro.2014.05.026

[115] Saris SC, Iacono RP, Nashold BS. Dorsal root entry zone lesions for post-amputation pain. Journal of Neurosurgery. 1985;**62**(1):72-76. DOI: 10.3171/jns.1985.62.1.0072

[116] Bouche B, Manfiotto M, Rigoard P, et al. Peripheral nerve stimulation of brachial plexus nerve roots and supra-scapular nerve for chronic refractory neuropathic pain of the upper limb. Neuromodulation: Journal of the International Neuromodulation Society. 2017;**20**(7):684-689. DOI: 10.1111/ner.12573

[117] Obiglio M, Mendelevich A, Jeffrey S, et al. Peripheral nerve stimulation effectiveness in the upper limb function recovery of patients with a stroke sequel: Systematic review and meta-analysis. Revista de Neurologia. 2016;**62**(12):530-538

[118] Johnson S, Goebel A. Long-term treatment of chronic neuropathic pain using external noninvasive external peripheral nerve stimulation in five patients. Neuromodulation: Journal of the International Neuromodulation Society. 2016;**19**(8):893-896. DOI: 10.1111/ner.12365

[119] Stevanato G, Devigili G, Eleopra R, et al. Chronic post-traumatic neuropathic pain of brachial plexus and upper limb: A new technique of peripheral nerve stimulation. Neurosurgical Review. 2014;**37**(3):473-479-480. DOI: 10.1007/s10143-014-0523-0

[120] Kim JH, Shin SH, Lee YR, et al. Ultrasound-guided peripheral nerve stimulation for neuropathic pain after brachial plexus injury: two case reports. Journal of Anesthesia. 2017;**31**(3):453-457. DOI: 10.1007/s00540-017-2315-5

[121] Van Calenbergh F, Gybels J, Van Laere K, et al. Long term clinical outcome of peripheral nerve stimulation in patients with chronic peripheral neuropathic pain. Surgical Neurology. 2009;**72**(4):330-335; discussion 335. DOI: 10.1016/j.surneu.2009.03.006

[122] Duncan CC, Kluger DT, Davis TS, et al. Selective decrease in allodynia with high-frequency neuromodulation via high-electrode-count intrafascicular peripheral nerve interface after brachial plexus injury. Neuromodulation: Journal of the International Neuromodulation Society. 17 Aug 2018. DOI: 10.1111/ner.12802. [Epub ahead of print]

[123] Linderoth B, Foreman RD. Physiology of spinal cord stimulation: Review and update. Neuromodulation: Journal of the International Neuromodulation Society. 1999;**2**(3): 150-164. DOI: 10.1046/j.1525-1403.1999.00150.x

[124] Wolter T, Kieselbach K. Cervical spinal cord stimulation: An analysis of 23 patients with long-term follow-up. Pain Physician. 2012;**15**(3):203-212

[125] Abdel-Aziz S, Ghaleb AH. Cervical spinal cord stimulation for the management of pain from brachial plexus avulsion. Pain Medicine (Malden, Mass.). 2014;**15**(4):712-714. DOI: 10.1111/pme.12313

[126] Deer TR, Mekhail N, Provenzano D, et al. The appropriate use of neurostimulation of the spinal cord and peripheral nervous system for the treatment of chronic pain and ischemic diseases: The Neuromodulation Appropriateness Consensus Committee. Neuromodulation: Journal of the International Neuromodulation Society. 2014;**17**(6): 515-550; discussion 550. DOI: 10.1111/ner.12208

[127] Haider S, Owusu-Sarpong S, Peris Celda M, et al. A single center prospective observational study of outcomes with tonic cervical spinal cord stimulation. Neuromodulation: Journal of the International Neuromodulation Society. 2017;**20**(3):263-268. DOI: 10.1111/ner.12483

[128] Piva B, Shaladi A, Saltari R, Gilli G. Spinal cord stimulation in the management of pain from brachial plexus avulsion. Neuromodulation: Journal of the International Neuromodulation Society. 2003;**6**(1):27-31. DOI: 10.1046/j.1525-1403.2003.03004.x

[129] Bennett MI, Tai YM. Cervical dorsal column stimulation relieves pain of brachial plexus avulsion. Journal of the Royal Society of Medicine. 1994;**87**(1):5-6

[130] Garcia-March G, Sánchez-Ledesma MJ, Diaz P, et al. Dorsal root entry zone lesion versus spinal cord stimulation in the management of pain from brachial plexus avulsion. Acta Neurochirurgica. Supplementum (Wien). 1987;**39**:155-158

[131] Dreval ON. Ultrasonic DREZ-operations for treatment of pain due to brachial plexus avulsion. Acta Neurochirurgica. 1993;**122**(1-2):76-81

[132] Prestor B. Microcoagulation of junctional dorsal root entry zone is effective treatment of brachial plexus avulsion pain: long-term follow-up study. Croatian Medical Journal. 2006;**47**(2):271-278

[133] Samii M, Bear-Henney S, Lüdemann W, Tatagiba M, Blömer U. Treatment of refractory pain after brachial plexus avulsion with dorsal root entry zone lesions. Neurosurgery. 2001;**48**(6):1269-1277

[134] Magistroni E, Ciclamini D, Panero B, Verna V. Ultrasound-guided pulse-dose radiofrequency: Treatment of neuropathic pain after brachial plexus lesion and arm revascularization. Case Reports in Medicine. 2014;**2014**:429618. DOI: 10.1155/2014/429618

[135] Ku B, Jun M, Lee J-H, et al. Short-term efficacy of pulsed radiofrequency thermal stimulation on acupoints for chronic low back pain: A preliminary study of a randomized, single-blinded, placebo-controlled trial. Evidence-Based Complementary and Alternative Medicine. 2018;**2018**:4510909. DOI: 10.1155/2018/4510909

[136] Boccard SGJ, Pereira EAC, Moir L, Aziz TZ, Green AL. Long-term outcomes of deep brain stimulation for neuropathic pain. Neurosurgery. 2013;**72**(2):221-230; discussion 231. DOI: 10.1227/NEU.0b013e31827b97d6

[137] Pereira EAC, Aziz TZ. Neuropathic pain and deep brain stimulation. Neurotherapeutics. Jul 2014;**11**(3):496-507. DOI: 10.1007/s13311-014-0278-x

[138] Levy R, Deer TR, Henderson J. Intracranial neurostimulation for pain control: A review. Pain Physician. 2010;**13**(2):157-165

[139] Aly MM, Saitoh Y, Kishima H, Hosomi K, Yoshimine T. Importance of distinction between paroxysmal and continuous patterns of pain during evaluation of pain after brachial plexus injury. Acta Neurochirurgica. 2011;**153**(2):437-438; author reply 439. DOI: 10.1007/s00701-010-0874-4

[140] Nashold BS. Current status of the DREZ operation: 1984. Neurosurgery. 1984;**15**(6):942-944

[141] Campbell JN, Solomon CT, James CS. The Hopkins experience with lesions of the dorsal horn (Nashold's operation) for pain from avulsion of the brachial plexus. Applied Neurophysiology. 1988;**51**(2-5):170-174

[142] Konrad P. Dorsal root entry zone lesion, midline myelotomy and anterolateral cordotomy. Neurosurgery Clinics of North America. 2014;**25**(4):699-722. DOI: 10.1016/j.nec.2014.07.010

[143] Chen HJ, Tu YK. Long term follow-up results of dorsal root entry zone lesions for intractable pain after brachial plexus avulsion injuries. Acta Neurochirurgica. Supplement. 2006;**99**:73-75

[144] Zhang X, Li Y, Hu Y, Tao W, Zheng Z. Dorsal root entry zone coagulation for treatment of deafferentation pain syndromes. Chinese Medical Journal. 2008;**121**(12):1089-1092

[145] Ruiz-Juretschke F, García-Salazar F, García-Leal R, et al. Treatment of neuropathic deafferentation pain using DREZ lesions; long-term results. Neurology (Barcelona, Spain). 2011;**26**(1):26-31. DOI: 10.1016/j.nrl.2010.10.003

[146] Tomycz ND, Moossy JJ. Follow-up 26 years after dorsal root entry zone thermocoagulation for brachial plexus avulsion and phantom limb pain. Journal of Neurosurgery. 2011;**114**(1):196-199. DOI: 10.3171/2010.5.JNS091520

[147] Thomas DG, Kitchen ND. Long-term follow up of dorsal root entry zone lesions in brachial plexus avulsion. Journal of Neurology, Neurosurgery, and Psychiatry. 1994;**57**(6):737-738

[148] Tasker RR, DeCarvalho GT, Dolan EJ. Intractable pain of spinal cord origin: clinical features and implications for surgery. Journal of Neurosurgery. 1992;**77**(3):373-378. DOI: 10.3171/jns.1992.77.3.0373

[149] Yoshida M, Noguchi S, Kuga S, et al. MRI findings of DREZ-otomy lesions. Stereotactic and Functional Neurosurgery. 1992;**59**(1-4):39-44. DOI: 10.1159/000098915

[150] Zheng Z, Hu Y, Tao W, Zhang X, Li Y. Dorsal root entry zone lesions for phantom limb pain with brachial plexus avulsion: A study of pain and phantom limb sensation. Stereotactic and Functional Neurosurgery. 2009;**87**(4):249-255. DOI: 10.1159/000225978

[151] Saris SC, Iacono RP, Nashold BS. Successful treatment of phantom pain with dorsal root entry zone coagulation. Applied Neurophysiology. 1988;**51**(2-5):188-197

[152] Chivukula S, Tempel ZJ, Chen C-J, Shin SS, Gande AV, Moossy JJ. Spinal and nucleus caudalis dorsal root entry zone lesioning for chronic pain: Efficacy and outcomes. World Neurosurgery. 2015;**84**(2):494-504. DOI: 10.1016/j.wneu.2015.04.025

[153] Stranjalis G, Torrens M. Dorsal root entry zone lesion performed with Nd:YAG laser. British Journal of Neurosurgery. 1997;**11**(3):238-240

[154] Levy WJ, Nutkiewicz A, Ditmore QM, Watts C. Laser-induced dorsal root entry zone lesions for pain control. Report of three cases. Journal of Neurosurgery. 1983;**59**(5): 884-886. DOI: 10.3171/jns.1983.59.5.0884

[155] Powers SK, Adams JE, Edwards MS, Boggan JE, Hosobuchi Y. Pain relief from dorsal root entry zone lesions made with argon and carbon dioxide microsurgical lasers. Journal of Neurosurgery. 1984;**61**(5):841-847. DOI: 10.3171/jns.1984.61.5.0841

[156] Young RF. Clinical experience with radiofrequency and laser DREZ lesions. Journal of Neurosurgery. 1990;**72**(5):715-720. DOI: 10.3171/jns.1990.72.5.0715

[157] Prestor B. Microsurgical junctional DREZ coagulation for treatment of deafferentation pain syndromes. Surgical Neurology. 2001;**56**(4):259-265

[158] Tomás R, Haninec P. Dorsal root entry zone (DREZ) localization using direct spinal cord stimulation can improve results of the DREZ thermocoagulation procedure for intractable pain relief. Pain. 2005;**116**(1-2):159-163. DOI: 10.1016/j.pain.2005.03.015

[159] Fazl M, Houlden DA, Kiss Z. Spinal cord mapping with evoked responses for accurate localization of the dorsal root entry zone. Journal of Neurosurgery. 1995;**82**(4):587-591. DOI: 10.3171/jns.1995.82.4.0587

Section 6

Challenges in Peripheral Nerve Surgery

Chapter 7

Starting A Peripheral Nerve Surgery Unit in an Area of Limited Resources - Our Experience

Chiazor U. Onyia, Ravi Sankaran and Ashok Pillai

Additional information is available at the end of the chapter

http://dx.doi.org/10.5772/intechopen.75349

Abstract

Dedicated peripheral nerve surgery centers are few in developing countries where majority of affected patients either remain untreated or are simply palliated with just physiotherapy. In this chapter, we review our experience with surgery for peripheral nerve lesions and peripheral nerve injuries over a 5-year period. A total of 68 procedures were carried out for 58 patients with various peripheral nerve lesions and injuries. Among the 19 surgeries for adult brachial plexus injuries, 10 were for pan-brachial plexus injury, 2 procedures for lower brachial plexus injuries, and 7 procedures for upper brachial plexus injury, while 11 repair surgeries were done for pediatric brachial plexus injuries. The remaining 38 surgeries included 21 peripheral nerve sheath tumor excisions, 5 ablative procedures for chronic neuralgia, 8 procedures for non-carpal tunnel peripheral nerve entrapments, and 4 adults with upper or lower limb isolated nerve injury repairs. The patients were followed up between 6 months and 2 years post-surgery for functional outcome assessment. Overall, as many as 57.5% of the patients had significant neurologic improvement noticed at 2 years of follow-up. Despite its challenges, optimal outcomes following surgery are still possible for patients with nerve injuries, entrapments, and nerve tumors in developing countries

Keywords: brachial plexus injury, peripheral nerve sheath tumor, peripheral entrapment neuropathy, pattern, peculiarities

1. Introduction

The field of peripheral nerve surgery has evolved significantly over the past century, with many lessons learnt [16]. The practice of peripheral nerve surgery can be both rewarding and frustrating due to prolonged recovery times and outcomes ranging from excellent to dismal, particularly for injuries involving the brachial plexus [44]. The most crucial aspect of planning surgical intervention in brachial plexus injury is selecting the timing of surgery [8]—preferably explored within 5 months after injury [8, 13]. This might be as early as 2 months for pan-plexus injuries which have demonstrated no improvement or as late as 5–6 months for distal neurotization repairs for upper plexus injuries. Generally, the armamentarium of the peripheral nerve surgeon includes (1) the initial history and examination, (2) preoperative electrophysiology, (3) preoperative rehabilitation, (4) longitudinal preoperative clinical and electrophysiological course (i.e., recovery/no recovery), (5) preoperative radiological assessment, (6) intraoperative anatomic study, (7) intraoperative electrophysiology, (8) operative procedures, and (9) postoperative rehabilitation.

However, this ideal kind of practice is obtainable mainly in the developed countries. Dedicated neurosurgical peripheral nerve surgery centers are still quite few in India and most other developing countries where majority of these patients either remain untreated or are palliated with physiotherapy as the only intervention, mainly as a result of lack of the required expertise and the necessary facilities. In this article, we looked at the pattern and trend of these problems in our practice, and present our early experience and outcomes, along with a brief review of previously documented results on similar surgical problems in the literature. Finally, we summarize the general principles and currently accepted practice guidelines required for optimal outcomes.

2. Patients and methods

The clinical and operative details of all patients who underwent peripheral nerve surgery at the neurosurgery department of Amrita Institute of Medical Sciences, Amrita University in Kochi, India over a period of 5 years from January 2010 till January 2015 were obtained from the hospital database and retrospectively reviewed. This department is a major neurosurgical referral center located in south-west of India serving both local and international patients. The senior author (AP) was responsible for the clinical and surgical management of all patients under review. The spectrum of cases ranged from nerve injuries and peripheral nerve sheath tumors to nerve entrapment syndromes. Short descriptions of the key approach and techniques which we used are briefly detailed as follows (with illustrations):

2.1. Nerve repair surgical technique

All our nerve repairs involved microanastomosis with 10.0 nylon epineural sutures (1–3 per coaptation) and fibrin glue, as described in the literature [45]. Our cable graft sources included the sural nerve, medial antebrachial cutaneous nerve (MACN), and occasionally the greater auricular nerve in infants. Some of our employed techniques for the extraplexal repairs included Somsak's selective distal neurotization of the axillary nerve with branch to long head of triceps [46], posterior approach and transfer of the spinal accessory nerve to the

http://dx.doi.org/10.5772/intechopen.75349

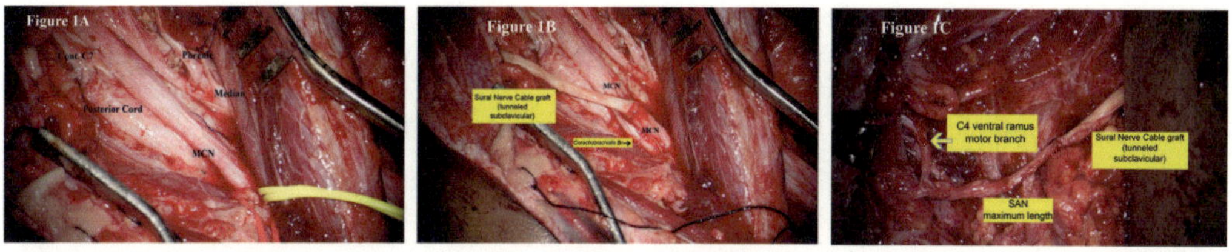

Figure 1. Intraoperative pictures of a sample extraplexal neurotization repair of pan-plexus injury. (A) Full-length phrenic nerve transfer to medial root of the median nerve for prehensile hand function and coaptation of contralateral C7 (Cont. C7) to the posterior cord for axillary and radial nerve functions. (B) Sural nerve cable graft in the same pan-plexus repair to neurotize the musculocutaneous nerve (MCN) from the spinal accessory nerve (SAN) for elbow flexion. The coaptation was made in the infraclavicular space into the MCN distal to the branch to the coracobrachialis. (C) Supraclavicular coaptation of ipsilateral C4 motor root and SAN as donor sources into sural nerve cable graft neurotizing the MCN.

suprascapular nerve for shoulder abduction, Oberlin I selective transfer of ulnar nerve fascicle to the musculocutaneous nerve and Oberlin II transfer of branch to brachialis with median nerve motor fascicle for elbow flexion [34]. Our extraplexal transfer techniques also used included contralateral C7 transfer with cable grafts tunneled through the prevertebral space (in 11 patients) to the posterior division of upper trunk for axillary and radial nerve reinnervation and/or the medial cord/branches in OBPI (obstetric brachial plexus injury) for hand function, and thoracoscopically harvested full length phrenic nerve transfer to medial root of median nerve for hand prehensile function (in 4 patients) (**Figure 1A–C**). Donor fascicle functional integrity and recipient nerve nonfunctionality was confirmed by the presence or absence of innervated muscle contraction in response to direct monopolar nerve stimulation. Post-operative immobilization of the affected limb was maintained for 3 weeks, and thereafter patients were commenced on a rigorous rehabilitation protocol by the second author (RS) as early as possible.

2.2. PNST (peripheral nerve sheath tumor) excision surgical technique

Under general anesthesia or regional anesthesia, the affected nerve segment was exposed, the epineurium was incised and tumor dissected in its subcapsular plane for PNSTs to ensure that non-involved fascicles remained functionally intact (**Figure 2c**). The entire limb was prepared and draped in order to assess all individual muscles with direct nerve stimulation as per the resection needs. Either direct NAP (nerve action potential) was recorded across the segment (2 cases) or absence of stimulation-induced target muscle twitching was ascertained before sacrificing the primary fascicle giving rise to the PNST. For malignant peripheral nerve sheath tumors (MPNSTs), an oncological wide resection at least 2–3 cm proximal and distal to the tumor, sacrificing the entire parent nerve, was done followed by functionally matched fascicular repair using sural nerve cable grafts (**Figure 3**). MPNSTs were often diagnosed preoperatively using FDG-PET (fluorodeoxyglucose positron emission tomography) scan to counsel and plan for nerve sacrifice and immediate repair.

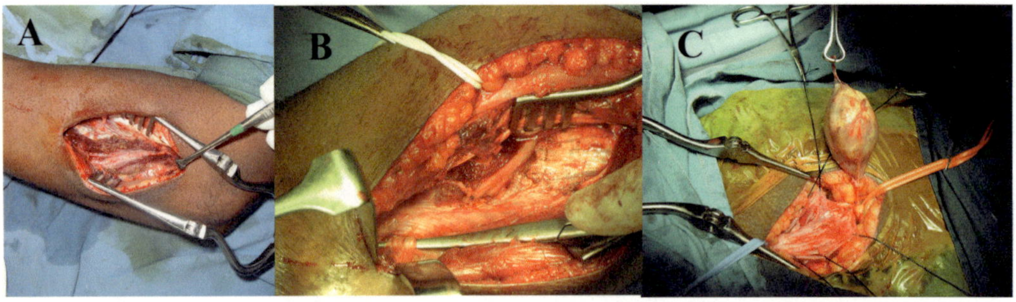

Figure 2. (A–C) Excision of a benign peripheral nerve sheath tumor. The affected nerve segment was first exposed, followed by incision of the epineurium and the tumor was then dissected out complete in its subcapsular plane.

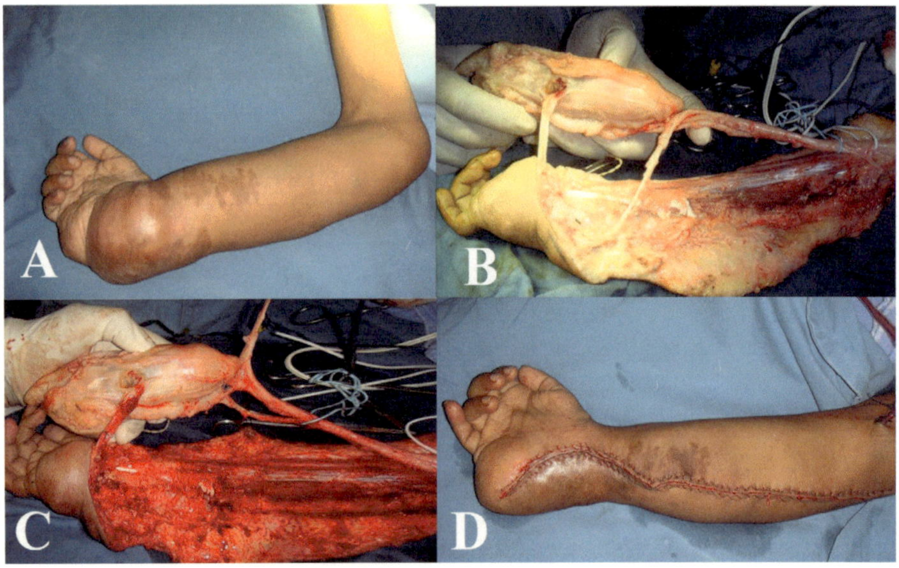

Figure 3. (A–D) Excision of a malignant peripheral nerve sheat tumor. Notice the extent of involvement of the affected limb. An oncological wide resection proximal and distal to the tumor was done along with excision of the involved parent nerve (C), followed by functionally matched fascicular repair using harvested cable grafts, as shown in (D).

2.3. Nerve entrapment release surgical technique

Nerve entrapments distal to the shoulder (cubital tunnel, PIN entrapment, Guyon's canal entrapment) were operated under regional (supraclavicular block) or local anesthesia. Previously described techniques were followed [1, 2, 21, 30] (**Figure 4A** and **B**).

Following surgery in each patient, the limb was immobilized with a splint for 2–3 weeks before commencing physiotherapy, to allow for epineural healing without tension at the anastomosis. Once the concerned limb was mobilized, our primary goals were prevention of contracture and prevention of complex regional pain syndrome (CRPS) following muscle reinnervation, by starting with passive ROM (range of motion). Once a flicker of contraction was found in the concerned muscles, we began isolating and strengthening them with gravity initially, progressing to "against gravity," and then with resistance. Once the patient could

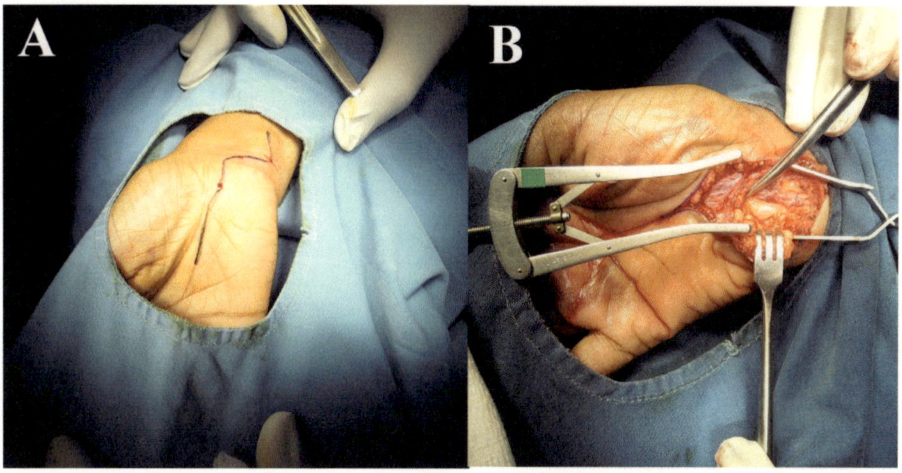

Figure 4. (A, B) Guyon's canal release. Notice the extent of the skin incision to both the wrist and palmar line (A) to ensure adequate exposure and release of the ulnar nerve and artery at the level of the canal.

move against gravity, it was useful to add functional tasks into the exercise programme since motor coordination is as important as strength in recovery. With this process, the patient would gradually develop "different" ways of doing old tasks to compensate for weakness of the primary effector muscle. This was achieved by utilizing the secondary effector muscles which changed the appearance of task performance.

If there was little hope of recovering function at this point, then focusing on stabilizing the involved muscles above and below became more practical but if the chances of functional recovery were high, then training the concerned muscle to become activated at the correct time in the kinetic chain became more useful than just purely strengthening it. Once the reinnervation waiting period was over, one of three patterns would usually emerge: (1) the patient recovered function in the limb and used it, (2) the nerve failed to reach and innervate the muscle, or (3) the reinnervation occurred but disuse would have reduced cortical representation and then, the patient may not know "how to" use the muscle. Electrophysiology was quite useful in differentiating such cases, and modifying the rehabilitation plan at this stage taken into consideration depending on which of these patterns was the case.

2.4. Outcome analysis

Our measurement of functional outcomes following surgery was defined as follows based on the Medical Research Council (MRC) motor power grading system [4, 20].

- No improvement in power = only flicker of movement of the affected muscle groups (or affected limb) = MRC 0–1
- Slight or mild improvement in power of affected muscle groups or the involved limb = MRC 2–3
- Significant improvement in power of affected muscle groups or the involved limb = MRC 4–5

The evaluations were carried out at 6 months, 1 year and 2 years after surgery at follow-up in our outpatient clinics.

3. Results

A total of 68 surgeries were completed in 58 patients for various peripheral nerve disorders over the 5-year period. There was an average of about 13.2 surgeries per year, with an increasing frequency as the programme developed. The age of the patients ranged from 2 month to 68 years, with a sex distribution of 41 males and 17 females (ratio of 2.4:1). Overall mean time of presentation was at 18.3 months either post-injury or following onset of symptoms for non-traumatic peripheral nerve problems, with the earliest presentation being 1 day post-obstetric brachial plexus injury in a newborn at birth and the latest being 15 years in 2 patients (one with a left ulnar nerve nodule and the other with a left brachial plexus PNST respectively). The majority of the cases were for brachial plexus injuries (n = 30, 44.1%) comprising 19 adult surgeries and 11 pediatric surgeries. Among the 19 adult surgeries, there were 10 procedures for pan-brachial plexus injuries, 7 for upper brachial plexus injuries and only 2 for lower brachial plexus injuries (**Table 1**). Of the 11 pediatric surgeries, 9 were for obstetric brachial pan-plexus injuries (OBPI—Erb's-Klumpke type) with one of the patients undergoing surgery twice while the remaining 2 were for road traffic accident traumatic injuries (**Table 1**). There were 21 excisions for peripheral nerve sheath tumors of which four were malignant, with one of these three patients requiring surgery twice (**Table 2**). There were 8 peripheral nerve entrapments comprising 3 posterior interosseous nerve entrapments, 3 cubital tunnel syndromes, 1 thoracic outlet syndrome and 1 Guyon's canal entrapment syndrome. The remaining 9 surgeries included repair for 2 patients with penetrating ulnar nerve injury, 2 patients with iatrogenic nerve injuries from PNST surgeries done elsewhere (brachial plexus and common peroneal respectively), and procedures for chronic neuralgia (which included 3 DREZ-otomies, image-guided radiofrequency lesioning, open neurotomy of lateral cutaneous nerve of the right forearm and selective fascicular neurectomy of the left distal ulnar nerve). Among the benign lesions, 12 (57.1%) were benign schwannomas, while the remaining 42.9% consisted of various other lesions. Of note, 3 patients undergoing PNST using the fascicular-sparing subcapsular dissection technique noted post-op sensory deficits or paresthesias which were generally transient and none was noted to have any motor deficits.

	n	Percentage
Pan-brachial plexus injury (adult)	9	30.0%
Upper brachial plexus injury (adult)	7	23.3%
Lower brachial plexus injury (adult)	2	6.67%
Obstetric brachial plexus injury (OBPI)	10	33.3%
Surgically managed Non-obstetric traumatic brachial plexus injuries	2	6.67%
Total	**30**	**100.0%**

Table 1. Distribution of surgery for adult and pediatric brachial plexus injuries.

As shown in **Table 3**, the majority of the injuries were repaired with various extraplexal neurotization transfers alone (25.8%), followed by repair with various combinations of extraplexal transfers and intraplexal neurotizations (22.6%), while 19.4% had repair with only intraplexal neurotizations. **Figure 5** summaries all surgeries done over the 5 year period. Brachial plexus

	n	Percentage
Peripheral nerve sheath tumors	21	55.3%
Peripheral nerve entrapments	8	21.1%
Chronic neuralgia	5	13.2%
Common peroneal nerve injury	1	2.6%
Ulnar nerve injury	3	7.9%
Total	**38**	**100.0%**

Table 2. Distribution of surgery for other lesions (adults and children).

	n	Percentage
Intraplexal neurotization	6	19.4%
Extraplexal neurotization/distal nerve transfers	8	25.8%
Combined intra + extraplexal neurotizations	7	22.6%
Exploration with internal/external neurolysis	3	9.7%
Microsurgical dorsal root entry zone lesioning (DREZ-otomy)	4	12.9%
Only microsurgical exploration + neurophysiological studies	3	9.7%
Total	30	100%

Table 3. Breakdown of all procedures done for brachial plexus injuries.

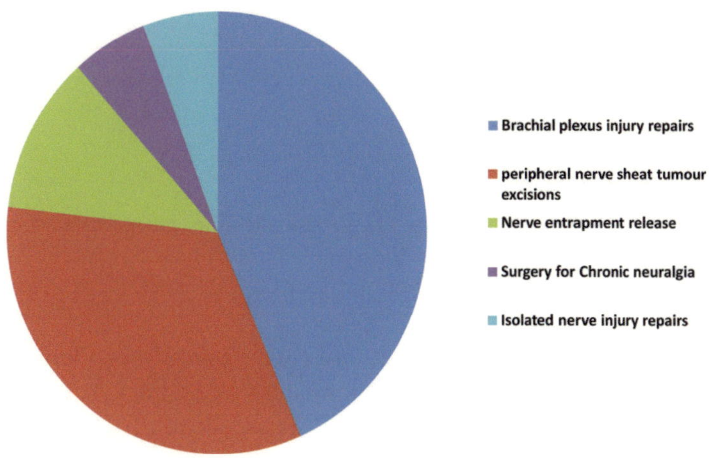

Figure 5. Summary of various peripheral nerve surgeries done over the five year period under review. Brachial plexus injury repairs and PNST excisions formed the bulk of the procedures.

	6 months post-op	1 year post-op	2 year post-op
N	19 (100%)	19 (100%)	18 (95%)
No improvements in function	12 (63.2%)	3 (15.8%)	—
Slight improvement	3 (15.8%)	7 (36.8%).	3 (15.8%)
Significant improvement	2 (10.5%)	5 (26.3%)	8 (42.1%)
No follow-up	2 (10.5%)	4 (21.1%)	7 (38.9%)

Table 4. Summary of outcomes for the adult brachial plexus injury repair.

	6 months post-op	1 year post-op	2 years post-op
N	11 (100%)	11 (100%)	10 (91%)
No improvements in function	3 (27.2%)	—	—
Slight improvement	4 (36.4%)	3 (27.2%)	—
Significant improvement	2 (18.2%)	5 (45.5%)	8 (72.8%)
No follow-up	2 (18.2%)	3 (27.2%)	2 (18.2%)

Table 5. Summary of functional outcomes for the pediatric brachial plexus injuries.

Complication	n	Percentage (%)
Voice hoarseness	2	13.3
Muscle weakness (post-PNST excision)	3	20.0
Operative wound dehiscence	2	13.3
Operative wound infection	3	20.0
Severe intra-op hemorrhage	1	6.67
Apnoeic attacks	1	6.67
Malunion (following claviculectomy for access)	1	6.67
Deep venous thrombosis of affected limb	1	6.67
Post-op pleural effusion	1	6.67
Total	15	100.0

Table 6. Post-operative complications.

injury repairs and PNST excisions formed the bulk of the procedures. Outcomes at 6 month, 1 year and 2 years post-op are as summarized in **Tables 4** and **5**. Complications following surgery are as shown in **Table 6**.

http://dx.doi.org/10.5772/intechopen.75349

4. Discussion

4.1. Perculiarities, trend, and pattern

Majority of the entire 58 patients were first seen at the out-patient clinic, while a few of them presented via the emergency room. Similar to observations in the literature, the more commonly affected anatomic side was the right side (58.5%) compared to 36.9% of the patients who had their problems on the left, with the remaining 4.6% who were mainly Neurofibromatosis-1 patients having bilateral PNSTs. There was a slight male preponderance of 2.4:1 in this study. Most other investigators similarly reported male predominance in their work (**Table 6**). From the observations as shown in the results, the majority of them were injury cases which were generally brachial plexus injuries (n = 30, 44.1%). Among the adult cases, pan-brachial plexus injuries were the commonest (n = 9; 50%), closely followed by upper brachial plexus injuries (n = 7; 38.9%) while lower brachial plexus injuries were the least (n = 2; 11.1%). Most of these presented fairly late (overall average time of presentation was 18.3 months) as a result of considerable length of time required for referral and transfer to our center following occurrence of the injury. As a result, majority of the procedures were done on elective basis instead of as emergencies. A few other factors which were probably responsible for late presentation possibly included poverty, living far away from our institution, initial visitation or consultation to other alternative healers, and sometimes delayed referral from other medical facilities. The follow-up rate at the end of the 2 year period was 95% for adults (**Table 4**) and 91% for the pediatric cases (**Table 5**) of the brachial plexus injury surgeries. The peripheral nerve sheath tumors ranked next in frequency (n = 21, 30.9%). The timing and pattern of presentation of this set of patients did not differ significantly from the nerve injury patients. Similar to the general pattern in the literature [14], the majority of the peripheral nerve tumors were benign. We had only 8 peripheral nerve entrapments while procedures for chronic neuralgia were the fewest (n = 3, 4.4%). Estimated blood loss was negligible in all surgeries except in one case of longstanding left brachial plexus PNST (**Table 6**). The post-operative complications noted in 22.1% of the patients post-operatively were mostly wound infection and post-PNST excision muscle weakness (**Table 6**).

4.2. Outcomes

Anyone would agree that timing of surgery is very crucial in the ultimate outcome. Yet, in spite of the fairly late presentation in the majority, it is clear from **Tables 4** and **5** that despite the relatively small number of 58 patients in our series, there was generally a steady rise in number of those with marked improvement of functional recovery, with a simultaneous decline in the proportion of "no improvements at all" over the same period. We did more of adult brachial plexus injury repairs and became less enthusiastic about pediatric cases as our practice developed because the adult cases generally benefitted from surgical repair (**Figure 6**). In our personal experience with managing 196 cases of Erb's and Erb's plus palsies, excellent recoveries were possible in majority of cases with just a proper rehabilitation programme consisting of cerebral retraining and judicious management of co-contracture deformities.

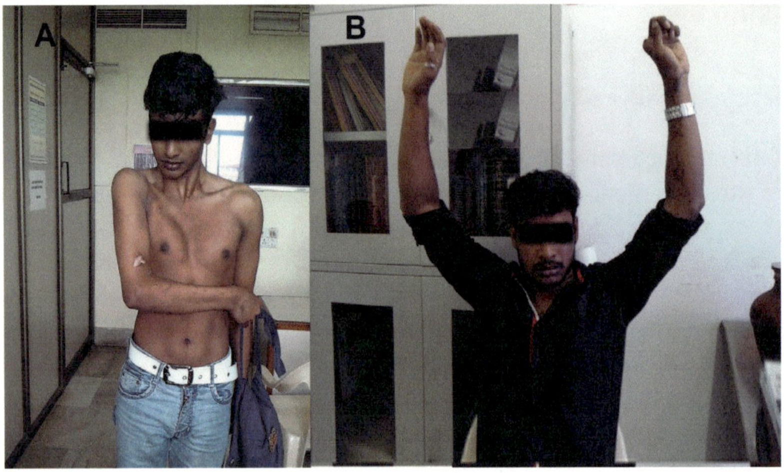

Figure 6. (A) Examination to evaluate function at 1 year post-op for extraplexal neurotization repair in a 19 year old male patient who had right brachial plexus injury involving upper and middle trunks. Notice the quite remarkable extent of power recovered particularly with elbow flexion. (B) Examination to evaluate function at 2 years after surgery for distal intraplexal neurotization repair in another 19-year-old male patient who had injury involving only the upper trunk of his right brachial plexus. Compared with the contralateral limb, he had recovery of power to almost the same level with the pre-morbid state.

4.3. Our challenges

Among those patients undergoing peripheral nerve procedures for pain, the outcomes were generally poor. The patient with painful neuralgia involving lateral cutaneous nerve of forearm responded only temporarily to two RF (radiofrequency) lesioning procedures, but was relieved completely by proximal neurotomy. However, the same patient eventually later developed another painful neuralgia from the medial antebrachial cutaneous nerve being entrapped in the previous neurotomy surgery scar. The patient who had selective ulnar fasciculotomy for left common palmar digital neuralgia experienced temporary relief for just 2 weeks, followed by recurrence of the same pain. Patients who had DREZ-otomy (dorsal root entry zone lesioning) had excellent initial relief with cessation of incapacitating pain attacks, but constant background neuralgic pain persisted with lesser severity than it was preoperatively. Additionally, for the brachial plexus injury patients, in spite of our meticulous techniques, the restoration of function below the elbow following either partial root avulsion or total root avulsion was our biggest challenge. The benefit of surgery over natural history was not also clear in the cases of OBPI, even despite the fact that only pan-plexus OBPI (Erb's-Klumpke type) were selected for surgical reinnervation. This explains why we did more of adult brachial plexus injury repairs and became less enthusiastic about pediatric repairs as the peripheral nerve programme went on.

Finally, among the several investigative imaging modalities required as standard pre-operative evaluation for peripheral nerve problems, one imaging modality which is emerging as a useful tool in preoperative selection and planning of peripheral nerve surgery is the MR neurogram [4, 41] but this was unavailable for investigating our patients at the time of their evaluation.

4.4. Steps followed in starting and organizing our peripheral nerve unit

One of the key aspects of the practice that can often lead to discouraging results if not properly addressed especially at the initially starting phase is how to select the right cases for surgery and get them properly managed after surgery. We realized that the ability of our efforts to manage these problems individually was limited. We constituted a multidisciplinary team comprising the neurosurgeons, neurologists, physiotherapists, orthopedician and plastic surgeon to review each patient and ensure adequate and appropriate pre-operative planning. The team met once a week and, this way, we were able to prevent the possibilities of inadequate or suboptimal clinical and electrophysiological localization/understanding of the process in each patient, know of any limitations of nerve repairs per case, plan ahead for accurate and reliable intraoperative electrophysiology as well as for reconstructive procedures at the muscle and tendon level. This arrangement also helped with meeting the need for regularized and effective rehabilitation as well as for motivation & consistent follow-up. At surgery, we utilized cable grafts as much as possible to prevention tension on our repair and made use of the operating microscope to ensure adequate microanastomosis. Interestingly, we did not have to advertise our work. There was already a strong referral pattern in our institution for other neurological/neurosurgical problems, and this was further consolidated for peripheral nerve related-problems by our multidisciplinary team. Regarding the problem of getting late referrals, we could only plan surgery based on how late the presentation was. Luckily, none of the patients in our series was too late on arrival as to benefit from only free muscle transfers. Unfortunately for most of such cases, we could not be in contact with the referring physician or health facility to ensure earlier referrals for subsequent cases.

4.5. Comparison with previous findings in the literature

Table 7 shows previous publications on surgery for various peripheral nerve problems and the documented outcomes. Reports from some of these studies highlight on a few technical factors positively influencing the results post-operatively. With respect to trauma, single coaptation repair of a donor nerve to the recipient nerve (neurotization repair) without tension is thought to be generally superior than indirect repair with a cable graft [13]. Bhatia et al., clearly demonstrated faster recovery and better functional results with direct coaptation compared to nerve graft interposition in carrying out contralateral C7 transfers while in a retrospective study on the effect of combining direct repair with nerve transfer procedures on the clinical outcomes in 74 patients by Sulaiman et al., all patients who had combination of nerve transfers with direct repair using either C5 or C6 recovered elbow flexion to Medical Research Council grade 3, compared to the same extent of recovery in only 87% of those in whom only nerve transfers were done [29, 36]. This further confirms the effectiveness of bypassing the long distance of regeneration by neurotizing the injured distal nerve stumps with more proximally located dispensable donor nerves [29]. In our experience however, though we did not do any comparative assessments like these authors, we attribute our outcomes as presented to the dedicated techniques and approach along with a strict rehabilitation program. We used combinations of cable graft techniques with direct neurotization transfers for majority of the brachial injury surgeries (**Table 3**) and for the functional priorities, elbow flexion and extension were generally the most important function of target we aimed to restore, closely followed by selective reinnervation of the median nerve for prehensile hand function or pincer grip.

Authors and year	No. of patients studied	Mean age	Sex distribution (M:F)	Type of lesion/ injury	Surgical techniques evaluated	Key results/outcomes	Maximum/mean follow-up
Guha et al. 2017 [35]	175	45.2 years	96:79	19 MPNSTs, 133 schwannomas, 49 neurofibromas	N/A	Less motor deficits with full resection of tumor; Increased recurrence with subtotal resections.	29.5 months
Bhatia et al. 2017 [36]	22	23 years for direct coaptation group; 24 years for nerve graft group	19:3	Brachial plexus injuries	Contralateral C7 transfer: By direct coaptation in 12 With graft interposition in 10	Direct coaptation group = Grade 3 flexion in wrist + fingers in 10; Grade 2 flexion in 2 Nerve graft group = Grade 3 flexion in wrist + fingers in only 2; Grade 2 flexion in 7; total failure in 1	26 months for direct coaptation group; 28.5 months for nerve graft group
Sulaiman et al., 2009 [29]	74	32 years	60:14	Brachial plexus injuries; tumor; irradiation	Medial pectoral to musculocutaneous N. transfers (Group 1); Intercostal to musculocutaneous N. transfers (Group 2)	Recovery of elbow flexion to MRC grade 3 in all (100%) who had both nerve transfer + direct repair with C5/C6 combined, but in only 87 and 22% of those who had only nerve transfers in Group 1 and Group 2 respectively	3.5 years
Badr et al., 2009 [4]	16	16 months	N/A	OBPI (2 Erbs, 6 Erbs plus, 8 Erb-Klumpke palsies)	Neurolysis; graft repairs; nerve transfers	Improvement from preoperative average biceps grade of 0 to 1/5 to average postoperative biceps grade of 2.9 and average shoulder abduction grade of 2.5	23.5 months
Sequeira and Martins, 2009 [27]	10	24.8 years	9:1	Complete brachial plexus palsy	Nerve transfers: phrenic to musculocutaneous N + spinal accessory to suprascapular N	Recovery to functional level in 7 (MRC Grade 3 in 5; Grade 4 in 2) No clinically significant respiratory problem in all 10 cases.	3.4 years

N/A, information not available; MPNSTs, malignant peripheral nerve sheath tumors; MRC, Medical Research Council; OBPI, obstetric brachial plexus injury.

Table 7. Previous publications on outcomes of various surgical techniques for peripheral nerve problems.

Regarding tumors, Guha et al., in managing 201 peripheral nerve sheath lesions (182 benign and 19 malignant) in 175 patients over a 17-year period, observed that subtotal resection was associated with the increased recurrence of the benign lesions and that the probability of motor function worsening postoperatively was much less in patients in whom the tumors were fully resected [35]. They also observed that the extent of resection in those who had schwannoma was greatly influenced by tumor location, with lesions located in the extremities being more likely to be fully resected than plexal tumors that were brachial, thoracic, or lumbosacral [35]. This was likely due to better anatomical accessibility [35]. They concluded by suggesting gross total resection for all benign lesions as much as possible [35]. In our own strategy however, we similarly dissected the tumor in its subcapsular plane for PNSTs to ensure that non-involved fascicles remained functionally intact but observed no recurrence of the benign lesions in any of our patients whereas oncological resection and not subcapsular dissection was our goal for the malignant ones (MPNST) in view of the life-threatening nature of the pathology, even at the cost of functional compromise.

4.6. General principles

Detailed examination of these patients should be followed up by nerve conduction studies and radiological imaging to localize and characterize peripheral nerve lesions or associated neurologic injury [3, 5, 8, 22]. The appropriate imaging modalities for evaluation should be selected depending on the particular clinical circumstance [3, 5, 8]. Plain-film X-ray, computerized tomography myelogram (CT), magnetic resonance imaging (MRI), ultrasound (US), as well as positron emission tomography (PET) all have their various indications in the management of peripheral nerve problems [3, 40]. For instance, transverse process fractures of the cervical vertebrae on cervical spine x-rays might indicate root avulsion at the same level [3, 22] and a distal neurotization repair can be preoperatively decided upon. CT myelography can be used to define the level of nerve root injury preferably within 4 weeks of the injury [3, 22]. Ultrasound may be used in some selected situations for localizing peripheral nerve entrapment and for image guidance in percutaneous interventions [3, 10]. One imaging modality which is emerging as a useful tool in preoperative selection and planning of peripheral nerve surgery is the MR (magnetic resonance) neurogram [3, 15, 37]. Of all these modalities, MRI and CT myelogram are generally the main radiological investigations for diagnosis of problems involving the brachial plexus [3, 5, 9, 37, 40].

Electrodiagnostic studies are equally essential, particularly electromyography (EMG) and nerve conduction studies (NCS). For example, preservation of sensory nerve action potentials (SNAPs) in extensive brachial plexus injuries with severe motor deficits is highly indicative of preganglionic injury and root avulsion. Additionally, serial compound motor action potential (CMAP) studies at 6 week periods give the surgeon an estimate of the spontaneous recovery potential of an injury (i.e., the classical neuropraxia and axonotmesis injury versus neurotmesis patterns) [18, 25]. When the electrophysiology findings are combined with the longitudinal clinical evaluation of motor recovery, the surgeon can then better decide upon timing and extent of repair required.

4.6.1. Brachial plexus injury repairs

Intra-operatively, the integrity of the donor nerve is a major determining factor for successful outcomes [13]. Single coaptation repair of a donor nerve to the recipient nerve (neurotization repair) without tension is generally considered superior to indirect repair with a cable graft, since only one microanastomosis is required [13, 45]. This is particularly important for weak donor nerves such as the spinal accessory nerve [13, 51]. According to functional priorities, elbow flexion and extension are generally the most important function to restore [19, 43]. Active shoulder control and stability is then considered next most important [50], followed by abduction, external rotation, wrist extension and scapular stabilization prioritized in that order [19]. Finally, managing each patient's expectations is perhaps the most important part of pre-operative planning and preparation [19]. Patients must be made to understand the limits of the best possible outcome and the possibility that either no improvement at all or limited functional improvement may occur after surgery [19].

The workhorse of brachial plexus repair surgery is still largely the neurotization transfers and nerve grafting [5, 6, 13, 17, 19, 23, 24, 29, 38, 42, 44, 48, 50, 51]. The muscles of the shoulder and the biceps brachii have classically been the main targets for repair of brachial plexus injuries [17, 29, 38, 48]. However, there is now more importance on equally focusing on restoring at least elbow extension for functionality and even newer attempts at selective reinnervation of the median nerve for prehensile hand function or pincer grip [33, 39, 42]. For proximal upper limb functions, the two most important distal transfers are neurotization of the suprascapular nerve with spinal accessory nerve through a posterior approach for shoulder abduction and Oberlin's double fascicular transfer of ulnar and median nerve fascicles to the biceps and brachialis branches of the musculocutaneous nerve for elbow flexion [8, 19, 23, 24, 26, 31, 33, 38, 47]. Case series reports have demonstrated very low long term donor nerve functional impairment resulting from thoracoscopic full-length phrenic nerve harvest and transfers and contralateral C7 transfer [8, 12, 13, 19, 27, 28, 33, 43, 44]. Our experience with these two procedures was very similar. Microsurgical dorsal root entry zone lesioning (DREZ) has been used to effectively control the intractable pain that follows brachial plexus injuries, particularly for the refractory cases [7, 11].

4.6.2. Nerve entrapments and painful neuropathies

For treatment of cubital tunnel syndrome, the anterior transposition of ulnar nerve may be done in either the subcutaneous or the intramuscular plane [30]. In situ decompression of the ulnar nerve with or without medial epicondylectomy as an alternative technique has also been well described with its pros and cons [30]. For patients with Guyon's canal syndrome, initial approach should be conservative care including immobilization, ergonomic modifications of habitual movement, and local injection of cortisone is advocated except for the refractory cases [2]. However, early motor involvement is common and one should then proceed to surgical decompression. At surgery, the skin incision should extend to both the wrist and palmar line, and the ulnar nerve and artery should be adequately freed at the level of the Guyon's canal [2] (**Figure 4A** and **B**). Posterior interosseous nerve (PIN) entrapment creates a functionally disabling pure motor deficit. For PIN release, the nerve must first be identified proximally between brachioradialis and extensor carpi radialis longus and distally between extensor carpi radialis brevis and extensor digitalis communis at the point where it enters the supinator, and should also include adequate division of the compressive supinator fibers.

4.6.3. Tumors

The goal of surgical intervention in PNST is excision of the tumor to alleviate the symptoms caused by neural compression without incurring a sensorimotor deficit [14]. In MPNST, however, oncological resection is the goal given the life-threatening nature of the pathology, even at the cost of functional compromise. In such situations, nerve graft repair can be planned preoperatively. General, regional or local anesthesia may be used [14]. For general anesthesia, anesthetist must avoid the use of muscle relaxants since these agents would ultimately prevent the use of intraoperative stimulation and monitoring [14]. The limb should be exposed so as to monitor the distal muscle response to fascicular stimulation (**Figure 3**). The incision should be made over the involved portion of the nerve starting from 2 to 4 cm proximal to and extending 2 to 4 cm distal to the tumor [14]. The probability of malignant degeneration of a PNST to MPNST should be assessed preoperatively by (1) size, (2) presence and character of pain, (3) radiological criteria (MRI, PET), and (4) the presence of type 1 neurofibromatosis (which has a 20% propensity for MPNST). If suspicion of MPNST is low, a subcapsular enucleation of the tumor mass (usually schwannomatous) offers the best chance of gross total excision with relief of compressive symptoms and simultaneous functional preservation of the nerve fascicles. However, when any combination of these features indicate high suspicion of an MPNST, thorough preoperative planning and counseling should be done for nerve sacrifice to maintain oncologically complete resection and subsequent grafting repair. Oncologically speaking, the option of initial tumor biopsy for confirming the histology followed by total resection is not ideal since violation of soft tissue planes leads to a higher chance for adjacent tissue seeding of sarcomatous cells and even delayed distant recurrence. If a nerve graft was done, the limb should be immobilized with a splint for 2–3 weeks to allow for epineural healing without tension at the anastomosis [14]. Fortunately, the majority of peripheral nerve tumors are benign [14].

4.6.4. Rehabilitation

Rehabilitation constitutes the remaining postoperative period until the patient achieves maximal functional and neurological recovery [49]. This can often be rather prolonged, and major depression related to extent of injury and surgery is a common factor that needs specific attention in order to improve outcomes. Once the concerned limb can be mobilized, the primary goals are prevention of contracture by passive ROM (range of motion) [41, 49]. This helps prevent complex regional pain syndrome (CRPS), and allows for a more useful limb once muscle reinnervation occurs. Within this time frame, orthotics is useful in preventing contractures at rest. This phase can extend up to 6–9 months post-operatively.

Once a flicker of contraction was found in the concerned muscles, we began isolating and strengthening them with gravity initially, progressing to "against gravity," and then with resistance. Once the patient could move against gravity, it was useful to add functional tasks into the exercise programme since motor coordination is as important as strength in recovery [41]. With this process, the patient would gradually develop "different" ways of doing old tasks to compensate for weakness of the primary effector muscle. This was achieved by utilizing the secondary effector muscles which changed the appearance of task performance. It remained with the physiotherapist to track recovery and see if these different ways were acceptable or not, followed by modification of the therapy plan as required. For example, the patient may develop "whip-like" movements to initiate shoulder abduction. If there was little hope of recovering deltoid function, then focusing on stabilizing the involved muscles above and below became more practical than utilizing electrical current to recover this muscle's mass. If the chance of functional recovery was high, then training the concerned muscle to become activated at the correct time in the kinetic chain became more useful than just purely strengthening it. Once the reinnervation waiting period was over, one of three patterns would usually emerge: (1) the patient recovers function in the limb and uses it, (2) the nerve fails to reach and innervate the muscle, or (3) the reinnervation occurs but disuse would have reduced cortical representation and then, the patient may not know "how to" use the muscle. Electrophysiology was useful in differentiating such cases, and modifying the rehabilitation plan taken into consideration depending on which of these patterns was the case.

5. Present challenges with peripheral nerve surgery

In spite of a growing number of good surgical alternatives currently available such as introduction of phrenic nerve transfer to medial root of median nerve for prehensile hand function, the restoration of function below the elbow following either partial root avulsion or total root avulsion presently remains the biggest challenge in brachial plexus surgery [8, 13, 25, 33, 39, 42]. Avulsion injuries from C5 to T1 have been shown to be amenable to restoration of good shoulder and elbow function, but the restoration of satisfactory distal function is still yet to be well demonstrated [8]. However, new techniques to circumvent this problem have recently been proposed [39, 42]. For the obstetric brachial plexus injuries, another particular challenge is the restoration of abduction and external rotation in the shoulder joint [18] which is largely limited due to developmental apraxia which occurs at a cerebral level.

Regarding investigation and preoperative planning, EMG and nerve conduction studies have their own limitations [18, 25]. EMG itself only reflects the function of the individual motor units in a nerve and not really that of the entire nerve or the cerebral retraining required to establish function [25]. Also, in severe cases with a flail anesthetic arm, the absence of SNAPs often clearly indicates damage to post-ganglionic elements but cannot exclude a mixed lesion with associated root avulsion [18].

Furthermore, there are currently only limited algorithms to guide the surgeon on carrying out nerve transfers [13, 52]. The choice of which transfer to utilize in each case is largely dependent on each surgeon's philosophy, knowledge and experience as well as patient-related factors, a clear understanding of the involved anatomy of the brachial plexus in each patient, what is uninjured and still viable for nerve transfer repair, as well as available facilities and equipment [8, 13, 52]. A combination of long and variable recovery periods, variable patterns of injury, individual patient recovery factors and lack of uniformity in rehabilitation all lead to the overall lack of objective evidence-based guidelines for management. For pediatric patients, the criteria and timing of surgical intervention also still remains controversial [4]. Some have used the absence of recovery of the biceps muscle or shoulder function by 3 months of age as the indication for surgery in obstetric brachial plexus injury (OBPI), while others use 4 months or even 9 months as the time limit [4, 32]. In our personal experience with managing 196 cases of Erb's and Erb's plus palsies, excellent recoveries were possible in majority of cases with a proper rehabilitation programme consisting of cerebral retraining and judicious management of co-contracture deformities. Some would argue that deformities are less common with early nerve repair in OBPI, but this is yet to be proven definitively.

Finally, even though microsurgical repair of nerve injuries has advanced significantly over time, satisfactory functional recovery still remains a challenge [29]. The ultimate goal of a nerve repair should be a functional improvement that creates satisfaction for the patient in his or her daily activities and occupation and not simple improvement in the muscle power grading. This requires dedicated efforts in physical, psychological and vocational rehabilitation. Augmentation of the paralyzed limb using reanimative muscle or tendon transfer surgeries by the plastic surgeon often improves outcomes. Hence, a multidisciplinary team is ideal.

6. Conclusion

In this chapter, we have described the pattern and trend of peripheral nerve problems in our practice, and presented our challenges and outcomes, as well as the steps we followed to organize our peripheral nerve unit, followed by a review of general guidelines and principles of care. Peripheral nerves related problems, are unfortunately only palliated in most developing countries across the world. Although our experience in surgically treating these problems is still developing and with the few limitations as presented, the final outcomes demonstrate that surgical intervention is still better than just palliative measures alone or even nothing at all. We could still manage the problems successfully with fairly good outcomes despite few setbacks such as late presentation of patients, as well as unavailability of full investigative imaging modalities required as standard pre-operative evaluation for peripheral nerve problems. We are hopeful that this brief presentation would be a useful impetus for the introduction, development and implementation of nerve surgery programmes in other developing countries around the world.

Competing interests

The authors declare that they have no competing interests.

Funding/material support

None.

Author details

Chiazor U. Onyia[1], Ravi Sankaran[2] and Ashok Pillai[3*]

*Address all correspondence to: brashok@aims.amrita.edu

1 Neurosurgery Division, Department of Surgery, Obafemi Awolowo University Teaching Hospitals Complex, Ile-Ife, Nigeria

2 Department of Physical Medicine and Rehabilitation, Amrita Institute of Medical Sciences and Research, Kochi, Kerala, India

3 Department of Neurosurgery, Amrita College of Medicine, Ernakulam, Kerala, India

References

[1] Abuelem T, Ehni BL. Minimalist cubital tunnel treatment. Neurosurgery. 2009;**65**:A145-A149

[2] Aguiar PH, Bor-Seng-Shu E, Fernando Gomes-Pinto F, Almeida-Leme RJ, Freitas ABR, Martins RS, et al. Surgical management of Guyon's canal syndrome—An ulnar nerve entrapment at the wrist: Report of two cases. Arquivos de Neuro-Psiquiatria. 2001;**59**(1):106-111

[3] Amrami KK, Port JD. Imaging the brachial plexus. Hand Clinics. 2005;**21**:25-37

[4] Badr Y, O'Leary S, Kline DG. Management of one hundred seventy-one operative and nonoperative obstetrical birth palsies at the Louisiana State University Health Sciences Center. Neurosurgery. 2009;**65**:A67-A73

[5] Bhandari PS, Sadhotra LP, Bhargava P, Bath AS, Mukherjee MK, Babu P. Current trends in the management of brachial plexus injuries. Indian Journal of Neurotrauma. 2008;**5**(1):21-25

[6] Bishop AT. Functioning free-muscle transfer for brachial plexus injury. Hand Clinics. 2005;**21**:91-102

[7] Bonilla G, Masi GD, Battaglia D, Otero JM, Socolovsky M. Pain and brachial plexus lesions: Evaluation of initial outcomes after reconstructive microsurgery and validation of a new pain severity scale. Acta Neurochirurgica. 2011;**153**:171-176

[8] Brophy RH, Wolfe SW. Planning brachial plexus surgery: Treatment options and priorities. Hand Clinics. 2005;**21**:47-54

[9] Carvalho GA, Nikkhah G, Matthies C, Penkert G, Samii M. Diagnosis of root avulsions in traumatic brachial plexus injuries: Value of computerized tomography myelography and magnetic resonance imaging. Journal of Neurosurgery. 1997;**86**:69-76

[10] Chien AJ, Jamadar DA, Jacobson JA, Hayes CW, Louis DS. Sonography and MR imaging of posterior interosseous nerve syndrome with surgical correlation. AJR. 2003;**181**:219-221

[11] Chen HJ, Tu YK. Long term follow-up results of dorsal root entry zone lesions for intractable pain after brachial plexus avulsion injuries. Acta Neurochirurgica. Supplement. 2006;**99**:73-75

[12] Chen L, Gu Y, Hu S, Xu J, Xu L, Fu Y. Contralateral C7 transfer for the treatment of brachial plexus root avulsions in children—A report of 12 cases. The Journal of Hand Surgery. 2007;**32**(1):96-103

[13] Chuang DC. Nerve transfers in adult brachial plexus injuries: My methods. Hand Clinics. 2005;**21**:71-82

[14] Dorsi MJ, Belzberg AJ. Peripheral nerve tumors of the extremities; in a. In: Quiñones-Hinojosa, editor. Schmidek and Sweet Operative and Neurosurgical Techniques—Indications, Methods and Results. 6th ed. Philadelphia: Elsevier Saunders; 2012. pp. 2319-2327

[15] Filler A. Magnetic resonance neurography and diffusion tensor imaging: Origins, history and clinical impact of the first 50,000 cases with an assessment of efficacy and utility in a prospective 5000-patient study group. Neurosurgery. 2009;**65**:A29-A43

[16] Friedman AH. An eclectic review of the history of peripheral nerve surgery. Neurosurgery. 2009;**65**(4):A3-A8

[17] Fournier HD, Mercier P, Menei P. Repair of avulsed ventral nerve roots by direct ventral intraspinal implantation after brachial plexus injury. Hand Clinics. 2005;**21**:109-118

[18] Harper CM. Preoperative and intraoperative electrophysiologic assessment of brachial plexus injuries. Hand Clinics. 2005;**21**:39-46

[19] Kline DG, Tiel RL. Direct plexus repair by grafts supplemented by nerve transfers. Hand Clinics. 2005;**21**:55-69

[20] Laurent JP, Lee R, Shenaq S, Parke JT, Solis IS, Kowalik L. Neurosurgical correction of upper brachial plexus birth injuries. Journal of Neurosurgery. 1993;**79**:197-203

[21] McCarthy MJ, Varty K, Bell PRF. Experience of supraclavicular exploration and decompression for treatment of thoracic outlet syndrome. Annals of Vascular Surgery. 1999;**13**:268-274

[22] Moran SL, Steinmann SP, Shin AY. Adult brachial plexus injuries: Mechanism, patterns of injury, and physical diagnosis. Hand Clinics. 2005;**21**:13-24

[23] Ray WZ, Pet MA, Yee A, Mackinnon SE. Double fascicular nerve transfer to the biceps and brachialis muscles after brachial plexus injury: Clinical outcomes in a series of 29 cases. Journal of Neurosurgery. 2011;**114**:1520-1528

[24] Ray WZ, Yarbrough CK, Yee A, Mackinnon SE. Clinical outcomes following brachialis to anterior interosseous nerve transfers—Report of 4 cases. Journal of Neurosurgery. 2012;**117**:604-609

[25] Robert EG, Happel LT, Kline DG. Intraoperative nerve action potential recordings: Technical considerations, problems and pitfalls. Neurosurgery. 2009;**65**:A97-A104

[26] Schaakxs D, Bahm J, Sellhaus B, Weis J. Clinical and neuropathological study about the neurotization of the suprascapular nerve in obstetric brachial plexus lesions. Journal of Brachial Plexus and Peripheral Nerve Injury. 2009;**4**:15

[27] Sequeira MG, Martins RS. Phrenic nerve transfer in the restoration of elbow flexion in brachial plexus avulsion injuries: How effective and safe is it? Neurosurgery. 2009;**65**:A125-A131

[28] Songcharoen P, Wongtrakul S, Spinner RJ. Brachial plexus injuries in the adult. Nerve transfers: The Siriraj hospital experience. Hand Clinics. 2005;**21**:83-89

[29] Sulaiman OAR, Kim DD, Burkett C, Kline DG. Nerve transfer surgery for adult brachial plexus injury: A 10-year experience at Louisiana State university. Neurosurgery. 2009;**65**:A55-A62

[30] Tang P, Plancher KD, Bishai SK. Anterior submuscular transposition of the ulnar nerve. Techniques in Orthopaedics. 2006;**21**(4):318-324

[31] Tung TH, Novak CB, Mackinnon SE. Nerve transfers to the biceps and brachialis branches to improve elbow flexion strength after brachial plexus injuries. Journal of Neurosurgery. 2003;**98**:313-318

[32] van Ouwerkerk WJR, van der Sluijs JA, Nollet F, Barkhof F, Slooff ACJ. Management of obstetric brachial plexus lesions: State of the art and future developments. Child's Nervous System. 2000;**16**:638-644

[33] Xu W, Lu J, Qiu Y, Jiang S, Xu L, Xu J, et al. Hand prehension recovery after brachial plexus avulsion injury by performing a full-length phrenic nerve transfer via endoscopic thoracic surgery. Journal of Neurosurgery. 2008;**108**:1215-1219

[34] Zhao X, Lao J, Hung L, Zhang G, Zhang L, Gu Y. Selective neurotization of the median nerve in the arm to treat brachial plexus palsy: Surgical technique. JBJS. 2004;**86A**:736-742

[35] Guha D, Davidson B, Nadi M, Alotaibi NM, Fehlings GM, Gentili F, et al. Management of peripheral nerve sheat tumours: 17 years of experience at Toronto Western Hospital. Journal of Neurosurgery. 2018;**128**(4):1226-1234

[36] Bhatia A, Doshi P, Koul A, Shah V, Brown JM, Salama M. Contralateral C7 transfer: Is direct repair really superior to grafting? Neurosurgical Focus. 2017;**43**(1):E3

[37] Upadhyaya V, Upadhyaya DN, Mishra B. MR neurography in traumatic non-obstetric paediatric brachial plexopathy. European Radiology. 2018;**28**(6):2417-2424

[38] Hu CH, Chang TN, Lu JC, Laurence VG, Chuang DC. Comparison of surgical strategies between proximal nerve graft and/or nerve transfer and distal nerve transfer based on functional restoration of elbow function: A retrospective review of 147 patients. Plastic and Reconstructive Surgery. 2018;**141**(1):68e-79e

[39] Wu X, Cong XB, Huang QS, Ai FX, Liu YT, Lu XC, et al. Transposition of branches of radial nerve innervating supinator to posterior interroseus nerve for functional reconstruction of finger and thumb in 4 patients with middle and lower trunk root avulsion injuries of brachial plexus. Journal of Huazhong University of Science and Technology. Medical Sciences. 2017;**37**(6):933-937

[40] Fuzari HKB, Dornelas de Andrade A, Vilar CF, Sayão LB, Diniz PRB, Souza FH, de Oliveira DA. Diagnostic accuracy of magnetic resonance imaging in post-traumatic brachial plexus injuries: A systematic review. Clinical Neurology and Neurosurgery. 2018;**164**:5-10

[41] Bains R, Kattan A, Curtis CG, Stephens D, Borschel G, Clarke HM. Active range of motion over time in patients with obstetrical brachial plexus palsy: A 10-year analysis. Journal of Hand Surgery Ameican. 2018;**43**(4):386.e1-386.e7

[42] Abou-Al-Shaar H, Karsy M, Ravindra V, Joyce E, Mahan MA. Acute repair of traumatic pan-brachial plexus injury: Technical considerations and approaches. Neurosurgical Focus. 2018;**44**(Suppl1):V4

[43] Li WJ, He LY, Chen SL, Lyu YW, Wang SF, Yong Y, et al. Contralateral C7 nerve root transfer for function recovery in adults: A meta-analysis. Chinese Medical Journal. 2017;**130**:2960-2968

[44] Mathews AL, Yang G, Wan-Chu Chang K, Chung KC. A systematic review of outcomes of contralateral C7 transfer for the treatment of traumatic brachial plexus injury: An international comparison. Journal of Neurosurgery. 2017;**126**(3):922-932

[45] Bahm J, Gkotsi A, Bouslama S, El-Kazzi W, Schuind F. Direct nerve sutures in (extended) upper obstetric brachial plexus repair. Journal of Brachial Plexus and Peripheral Nerve Injury. 2017;**12**(1):e17-e20

[46] Jácome DT, de Alencar HFU, de Lemos MVV, Kobig RN, Rocha JFR. Axillary nerve neurotisation by a triceps motor branch: Comparison between axillary and posterior arm approaches. Revista Brasileira de Ortopedia. 2018;**53**(1):15-21

[47] Chang KWC, Wilson TJ, Popadich M, Brown SH, Chung KC, Yang LJS. Oberlin transfer compared with nerve grafting for improving early supination for neonatal brachial plexus palsy. Journal of Neurosurgery. Pediatrics. 2018;**21**:178-184

[48] Murison J, Jehanno P, Fitoussi F. rve transfer to biceps to restore elbow function and supination in children with obstetrical brachial plexus palsy. Journal of Children's Orthopaedics. 2017;**11**:455-459. DOI: 10.1302/1863-2548.11.170125

[49] El-Shamy S, Alsharif R. fect of virtual reality versus conventional physiotherapy on upper extremity function in children with obstetric brachial plexus injury. Journal of Musculoskeletal & Neuronal Interactions. 2017;**17**(4):319-326

[50] Vanaclocha V, Herrrera JM, Rivera-Paz M, Martinez-Gómez B, Vanaclocha L. Radial to axillary nerve transfer. Neurosurgical Focus. 2018;**44**(Suppl 1):V1

[51] Bulstra LF, Rbia N, Kircher MF, Spinner RJ, Bishop AT, Shin AY. Spinal accessory nerve to triceps muscle transfer using autologous long nerve grafts for recovery of elbow extension in traumatic brachial plexus injuries. Journal of Neurosurgery. Dec 8, 2017:1-7

[52] Pondaag W, van Driest FY, Groen JL, Malessy MJA. Early nerve repair in traumatic brachial plexus injuries in adults: Treatment algorithm and first experiences. Journal of Neurosurgery. Jan 26, 2018:1-7